The Last Diet Book You're Going to Ever Need: Break Stalled Weight-Loss with a Belly-Fat Melting Plateau Shattering Fiery Tea

Copyright ©2017 Trena Stevens

Editor: Irena Harold

Table of Contents

Medical Disclaimer

This book nor the author seeks to diagnose, treat illness or give advice to anyone seeking treatment for any kind of health condition. Anyone reading the information in this book should take this account as a personal story, which the author is sharing with the intention of inspiring other seekers to develop their own solution in collaboration with their own professional or medical healthcare provider or team. The author is not a medical professional and has no qualification as a licensed medical expert. NEVER DISREGARD PROFESSIONAL MEDICAL ADVICE or delay seeking medical attention because of something you've read or accessed through this book. You are encouraged to confirm any information obtained from this book with other sources and review all information regarding any medical condition or treatment with your physician. Neither the author nor the publisher shall be liable or responsible for any loss or damage allegedly arising from any information or suggestions in this book.

Acknowledgements

I thank God for the wonderful gift of this tea recipe. For reminding us that He has already provided everything that we need, that the major cause of our many illnesses is overindulgence and that it's never too late to make the changes necessary for a better quality of life.

To my family, church family and networking family-- for all you have done for me-- I thank you. Special thanks to my parents, Emerson and Irene Smith and James and Leah Harold for their support. To my husband, Kenneth E. Stevens, Sr.—love you Deacon Honey! To my daughter, Irena and grandson, Jordan and son Kenny Jr., I say thank you. To my sister in law, Rochelle Johnson-Smith—author of *T.R.U.T.H, The Rough Underlying Trials of Healing*, thank you for spurring me along and providing the connections to get this book accomplished. Special thanks to my brother Jimmy Harold for sharing his story about reversing his diabetes and sharing the concept of workout intensity. I want to especially thank my pastor, Rev. Dr. F. J. Alexander and his lovely wife, Brenda, along with the Sports and Health Ministry and each member of Philadelphia Missionary Baptist Church of Kirby, Texas.

Introduction

We all *know* what to do—decrease food intake and increase physical activity-- to lose the excess weight, get fit and be healthy. But it's determining how much to decrease in calories and increase in exercise AND *doing* it **CONSISTENTLY** *forever* that's problematic. How do we make fitness a permanent transformational (no going back) change for life? That's what I'd like to help you address through this book and the use of the tea recipe enclosed.

One real issue is that weight loss information tends to be thrown at us in a one-size-fits-all fashion when we each have individual needs. For example, we know that we need to eat right, but how strict or lenient we need to be depends on the person—starting weight, age, and whether male or female. We need to exercise but the type of exercise, length of time and intensity required to make a difference, also depends on the person. So there needs to be an individualized plan. A plan in which I'll give you a point of reference to start at the end of this introduction. Then as I share my story you can take a look at the different aspects of fitness that I went through; think about what the different meal plans and workout programs would mean to you; determine whether or not they will work for your purposes; and finally come to some agreements about incorporating them into your life real-time for genuine results.

Another issue is that *IT'S A MATTER OF CHEMISTRY.* Growing up what I loved the most about science was the experiments. However judging by the fact that you're reading this book, you're done with experimenting. So in this case I'll give you some tried and true actionable items. Where the experimental part comes in is that you need to try them to figure out which ones bring the right reactions to cause you to lose the *most* weight. Sometimes trials help, sometimes we get mixed results and other times they just do not work for us. A trial can be helpful because we are supplying ourselves with different spices, herbs, frequencies of eating, vitamins, supplements, different food and nutrient combinations and then different styles of exercising, etc. And if it is exactly what was needed we get good results. We often get mixed results because we are operating on abbreviated information. So when we hear about a tip or read an article, we need to go to the source just to make sure we are not missing vital information which can culminate into unsatisfactory results. Sometimes we cut ourselves short because we just do not try a new thing long enough for a difference to show up. Other times we see no difference. When this happens, there's no need to panic. It just means the trial didn't provide what was needed for weight loss. There will be times when we become frustrated if we fail to get the same results as others. That's why I suggest looking at it from a scientific point of view. As you may recall in science we develop a hypothesis, (something that we think is true) then we test it; to see if it is, in fact, true. So it is the same here, except you're trying different processes to see if they are, in fact, true for you—personally. If we go in with a trial and error approach and have the understanding that we're on a discovery mission then there's a better chance of leaving the emotions out of the equation. Then we suffer less of a setback in unfruitful trials. **When we do not get the expected results we have to go back and trace our steps.** For example, if the plan was to cut back 500 calories per day we should lose 1 pound a week but if due to miscalculation the items we cut from our food list actually total 300 calories instead of 500 calories per day; we'd have a better understanding of why we didn't get the desired results and could resolve to fix the issue. If we had a plan to increase our activity to burn 500 intentional calories per day outside of what we normally use in a day, we should lose a pound per week. But if we mistakenly chose an activity which actually burned an extra 300 calories per day instead of 500, we'd know what correction to make. Food for thought, if we were to reduce calories AND increase exercise and create a plan to run both of these trials at the same time we could expect to lose 2 pounds per week; plus we'd have a little wiggle room. We wouldn't have to be so exact because even if we made the same mistakes as in the previous examples, we'd lose at least 1 pound per week; which is at least some progress. If we follow a trial to the letter and fail to get good results, we can either modify the attempted system to fit our personal needs or choose a different one altogether. The key is to **KEEP TRYING** different ones until we find out what works best. We simply cannot afford to quit or get bent out of shape when we try something that doesn't work for us. Also, what you start out doing to bring the weight down is not likely to be how you'll finish when you reach your goal weight or, ultimately what you'll have to do to maintain it. The reason for that is that as your body changes there will be different requirements to keep the weight falling.

So then how can I be so certain that this book will be your last diet book? I'm going to help you get an understanding of weight-loss chemistry, give you the tools to use to your advantage and take the guess work out of it, but you're going to set your own eating boundaries and workout regimens. I'm going to help you only make agreements that you know you can keep because when you set your own rules; you have a better chance of keeping them. I'll give you the formulas and help you calculate the numbers so that you can get the scale moving in the right direction. I'll also show you a process so that you can graduate to lean eating rather trying to go lean, all at once—like a smoker trying to quit cold turkey. I want you to think about changing your point of view. I want you to no longer focus on back sliding, will power collapses and broken commitments. From now on I want you to focus on what you *can* do. And you'll be successful this time because you decide what you're willing to commit to, to reach your goals.

So the journey to fitness should not only be individualized and forged with an understanding of chemistry, but it should involve strategic development—which is setting plans into place to reduce resistance, opposition and barriers to change. Often people who are trying to lose weight will find something that works, but the issue is that old habits don't just go away; and neither do they take kindly to being de-throned. So the old ways are always looking for opportunities to rule again. Then it becomes extremely important to look at your old habits as a living, breathing branch of yourself that needs to be pruned. It will behoove you to plan ahead to make new habits stick. I'll help you learn to pinpoint the intersections where the new habit is to replace the old. Then I'll help you develop some strategies to avoid pitfalls of reverting to old ways by having the new ways ready to be practiced and reinforced. Therefore making you successful because you will have put into place new ways that are just as easy to choose over old ways. It really comes down to making the new plan a part of your new lifestyle.

Speaking of new lifestyle, that is exactly what you will be doing— creating a new one. You can't expect to *want* something different yet you, yourself, remain the same. You must change. You must do so—inside out, for change to be long lasting. Of course, there's not enough room in this book for psycho analysis but I found that there was a need to include a few chapters—Grow your Way Out, Beware of Dream Killers, Mental Strength, Faith and New Beginnings to devote to total wellness. It's important for you to consider making changes in your relationships with yourself, work, family, friends, food and physical activity and so on, to be successful in this process. You'll really want to concentrate on changing the conversations you have with yourself, loving yourself and being whole. As Mike Robbins stated, in his book entitled **Nothing Changes until You Do: A Guide to Self-Compassion and Getting Out of Your Own Way,** "The most essential human relationship we have is with ourselves." He contended that, "The more unhealthy and critical our relationships are with ourselves, the more it manifests in various negative ways in our lives. We sabotage our success; turn to addictions of all sorts (food, work, alcohol, drugs, sex, technology and so on)." He also heralds a solution, ***"Making peace with ourselves is fundamental to everything that truly matters in life."*** (Robbins, 2014). If you really dig deep, you'll be creating a whole new you. You're going to stretch yourself out so far that there's no way you can ever go back to the old you; which is neither fast nor easy.

Fast and easy, is another mistake we make. We think we can do this quickly. There is no fast and easy way to transform. It's a growing process because we have to expand our minds beyond what we currently know. It's also a two part process, we have to learn it and then we have to apply it. We *GO BEYOND* what we know by APPLYING that which we have learned. That was my issue. I was forever picking up a book, reading articles and studying every bit of research and trying to break down every report available to figure out what it all meant for me. All of it for naught because I wasn't putting into action any of the things I'd been reading because they were beyond what I could commit to doing. It never dawned on me to start where I was rather that start where I want to end up, until one day I read a book about habits called **Mini Habits: Small Habits, Bigger Results**, by Stephen Guise, I call him the one push-up guy. He had decided to work out and at the appointed time, to his disappointment, he found himself doing none of the things he'd set out to do. He was like I was— something he called "unstartable". I refer to it as a gap of unprepared strategy at the intersection of old habit versus new habit. To get past it he found one small thing that he could do to which his mind would raise no objection—one push up. That one push up turned into 15, and so on. So here's your first tool when you find yourself "unstartable" at the intersection of old habit and new habit, CHOOSE ONE SMALL, NON-THREATENING THING YOU *CAN* DO… AND DO IT… REPEATEDLY and keep doing it until it grows into a new habit. (Guise, 2013)

So as I share with you my story, I'm hoping it will help you make some decisions about what will work for you or at least what you want to try next. I hope to make the weight loss seem to go quickly with a provision of tools advantageous for determining the right food intake-to-activity ratio that will cause weight reduction to be more intentional.

There's a lot involved in regards to losing weight. There are just no short cuts if you want the required change to be perpetual. But if I could do it, you can too. Through growth and maturity, I learned a great deal in getting to where I am today—and I'm choosing to share it all with you. I've lost 40 pounds and I've kept it off a full year. This was something I'd never been able to do previously. Although I still have a long way to go, I have stopped the yo-yo dieting by mindful eating, developing some strategies to help me keep my commitments and by breaking the chains of my addiction to refined sugar. But most of all I learned to make a warm, tasty, fiery tea that melted the belly fat right off of me. I also use this tea whenever I hit a plateau. I drink the tea for 7 days straight and it helps me break through every time. This is my story about how the tea recipe has helped me overcome the challenges of weight loss.

You may be like I was with more than 20 pounds to lose, having the ability to stick to a diet and exercise plan for a short period of time like 3 to 4 weeks and lose 20 pounds. Only to hit a plateau, become discouraged and gain it all back and then some. I'm certain I've lost 20 pounds over 200 times before I found the tea. The tea recipe is what helped me get further than ever before. If this is you, you need to consider this recipe.

You may be on your last 20 pounds, so I do not have to warn you about plateaus. It's like anything else. The closer you get to your goal, the greater the challenges are to reach completion. The more exact you will have to be. This means less room for slacking off on your eating or exercise plans. You must change your routine (food as well as exercise) because your body has gotten used to what you've been doing. It takes a little more inertia and usually involves adding resistance, weights and or high intensity interval training (1 to 3 minute bursts of intensifying the activity and getting the heart rate up within a 20 to 30 minute routine) to reach a fat-burning state. You may consider going leaner in your meal plan—if that's possible. Make sure you're getting enough water. More than that, make sure you're getting enough overall calories per day, especially protein, fiber and good fats. Many people decrease their caloric intake too low, as mentioned in the chapter, So Sick of Eating I Didn't know What to Do and end up with a weakened body instead of a strong, fat-burning body. You may consider exercises that use the whole body (kettle bell or burpees) or within your normal routine you could do short focused work outs working different muscles than the ones you usually focus on. There was a time that I had to break up my 1 hour workout routine into three 20 minute-workouts (with high intensity bursts) per day to break a plateau. So variation is key and of course you'll want to also consider the tea recipe to help you break through.

Wherever you are in your fitness journey, you might be in need for this tea recipe as a good way to either jump start a plan and or obliterate plateaus. I'm hopeful that the exercises at the end of the chapters can help you make some agreements about which route you want to take. I hope to assist with techniques that will help you keep those agreements.

I think you should also note that I discovered that the tea helps whether you are trying to lose weight or not. When I shared the recipe with my husband, I was astonished that he achieved similar results with one week on the tea without being on any type of weight-loss program at all. He liked the results so well that he started taking the tea two times a day and his results increased exponentially. We did not see any more results beyond two weeks.

When family and friends started asking what I was doing to get my weight down, I told them about the tea and many asked for the recipe. When I started getting multiple requests for the recipe, that's when I knew that not only had God shown me what was missing from my weight loss plan, but that there was a need to get the information communicated and it has changed my life to be an instrument of healing. There was no way I could go without sharing it to help others. So I thought to put the recipe down in writing. As I recorded the recipe I realized that I needed to tell the whole story in order to do the most good. Then folks mentioned that it was a chore to get all the ingredients and make the recipe, I started making the base for people. And when that became cumbersome for me, I started making tea bags—Trena Tea, to which only the oils, lemon juice and apple cider vinegar have to be added.

My one true prayer and the purpose of this book is that in sharing my story you, too, may discover the missing pieces of your weight-loss puzzle to help you become a healthier you. Next you will find a grocery list, recipe and tips. Then I share my story as I flittered around from one stage to the next on this journey. I utilize the end of each section to help you hone in on the most important action items through exercises that prompt reflection to help you gain some leverage in this battle. And it is just that, a battle. So let's end this chapter with an actionable item that you can add to your arsenal—right now, today.

So let's cut a quick 500. Let me give you the background story first, then I'll give you the instructions. One day I was reading an article on My Fitness Pal.com that mentioned Michael Haub, a nutrition professor at Kansas State University. Being overweight, he put himself on a predominantly snack food diet known as the "Twinkie Diet" because Twinkies were the prominent part of the plan. He ate two Twinkies every three hours; what amounted to a vegetable plate for dinner (mostly green beans); a multi-vitamin; and a protein drink daily but excluded meat, grains and fruit from his diet. He lost 27 pounds in 10 weeks. Lowering his Body mass index (BMI) from 29 to 25, which was to go from almost obese to normal. His LDL (bad cholesterol) lowered and his HDL (good cholesterol) went up. Of course he doesn't condone such a dreadful diet and neither do I, but he did make the point that by going from 2600 calories per day to 1800 calories per day he lost weight. Regardless of the make-up of those 1800 calories-- (Twinkies, nutty bars and powdered donuts) he lost 27 pounds. I was overjoyed with that tidbit of knowledge. He was able to lose weight because he reduced his caloric intake BUT he was able to do so without them being all LEAN CALORIES—which was the major reason I hadn't been able to remain consistent. I had trouble sticking to a lean diet all the time. The article went onto explain that it takes a reduction of 500 calories per day over a 7 day period to lose a pound of fat. (Park, 2010) Instead of reducing my daily caloric intake all the way down to 1200 per day (average weight loss goal for women)-- a commitment I could not keep any way; I could back off 500 calories from my usual intake of 3000 per day to lose a steady pound of fat per week and keep reducing in increments of 500 until I was within the desired 1200 calorie per day range. So I began to formulate a plan to do a modified version of this plan to suit me. I very quickly chose a couple items that I could live without to strike from my list of foods. I decided to have coffee instead of my usual Frappuccino and eat one taco instead of two for breakfast. Further, I then made the decision that I wouldn't give up my favorite foods unless it got to the point that continuing to indulge impeded my progress. I sought ways to reduce my favorites down to 150-200 calorie servings. If I wasn't able to do that; I found ways to cut back elsewhere in my meal plans or workout more so that having a treat didn't ruin my weight loss plan. I was also grateful to have the knowledge to look over my food and exercise regime throughout a 7 day period and make adjustments to prevent a splurge from undermining my ultimate goals. So now it's your turn.

Cut a Quick 500 Exercise

1.   Make a list of what you generally eat in a week or if you have a food journal use a week that closely details what you typically eat.

2.   Next to each item write down the caloric value.

3.   Decide which items you can eliminate from the foods you eat right now, without heartburn. Strike as many as you can from your list, but make sure you're reducing at least 500 calories per day, minimum. This should create the 500 calorie deficit required to lose one pound per week. When you stop losing 1 pound per week, find 500 more pounds to eliminate from your diet.

As stated, I swapped a 510 calorie frozen coffee for a 95 calorie coffee with hazelnut cream; and cut another 250 calories by dropping down to one taco instead of two. This came to a 665 caloric intake deficit in looking at just one meal.

It was easiest for me to choose breakfast to find 500 calories to eliminate quickly because I ate the same thing every morning—Frappuccino and two tacos.

I wasn't ready to change anything else so I only changed breakfast. But this small change yielded a huge payoff. When I stopped getting results from that swap, I looked at my in between meals. I swapped my usual snack of a Grab Bag sized Cheetos® and a sweet tea or a Snickers® bar with a variety box of 100 calorie snacks and water. And so on; each time progress slowed, I reduced my caloric intake by 500 calories.

Before	Cal	Alternative	Cal	Deficit
Brkfst				
Frappe	510	Lg Coffee	95	415
2 tacos	500	1 taco	250	250
				—
				665

If you have greater variation in the things you eat from day to day it may be more difficult to determine what you will cut, but you can do it. Start by choosing the meals where you tend to eat the same things most days and see if you can make them 500 calories lighter. Next, make your snacks lighter by having fruits instead of candy, nuts and Skinny Girl® or Smartfood® popcorn instead of chips. Then try making water your go-to drink. Another thing you can do, consider choosing one meal of the day in which no matter what you eat, you agree to make it 500 calories lighter than what you normally do. Like I did when I finally wanted to have a better lunch. I knew that if I went into the cafeteria at work or out to lunch I wouldn't eat light; so I started bringing my lunch (usually two meat, cheese and spinach roll ups) to ensure that it was 500 calories lighter than usual.

(It was probably 1000 calories lighter than usual because my usual lunch was a bacon cheeseburger with fries; or two slices of pizza; or chicken fried steak with mashed potatoes and gravy; or enchiladas with rice and beans—well you get the idea.) Last but not least, one thing that goes a long way is to cut back on liquid calories. A 32 oz. soft drink has 420 calories but a 20 oz. soft drink has 240 calories especially if you ask for light ice like I used to do. At most places a large drink is 32 oz. Let's say you have three sodas per day and reduce from 32 oz. servings to 20 oz. servings you would create a deficit of 540 calories (180 x 3). Ask yourself do you really need a liter of soda to go with this one meal? If you bought a 2 liter bottle you'd drink 16 to 20 ounces at a time, so why drink 32 or 44 ounces of soda with one meal?

4.   Leave any items in your meal plan that stir up anxiety when you think in terms of giving them up. Instead of giving them up totally, think about having smaller portions or lighter versions.

5.   For the items that you do not intend to give up, count up the cost. Get an understanding of what this indulgence means to your ability to create a 500 calorie deficit per day. What I mean is know how much exercise or cutting back elsewhere on other food intake it takes to zero the item out. **For example my favorite treat is a 380 calorie, Dairy Queen Reese's Peanut Butter Cup Blizzard Mini. So when I have this treat I know that it comes with**

giving up two, 150 calorie snacks and running an extra mile during my workout.

6. **Calculate your physical activity.** *To calculate your total calorie burn per mile of WALKING, multiply your weight by .53. So as a 200 pound person I would burn 106 calories per mile so I could do an extra mile per day for 4 days if I decided to zero it out with exercise only.*

To calculate your total calorie burn per mile RUNNING, multiply your weight by .75 which would mean a 150 calorie burn for a person weighing 200 pounds and a 131 calorie burn for a person weighing 175 pounds. (McDougall, 2015)

Quick 500 Journal

List what you typically eat in a day along with their caloric value, then choose some items to strike

Breakfast____

____

Snack____

____

Lunch____

____

Snack____

____

Dinner____

____

Snack____

____

____

Twist on Professor Haub's Plan

1.	My twist on Professor Haub's plan is 1 protein drink, 2 snacks and 2 meals. My eating times are every three hours-- 8 am, 11 am, 2 pm, 6 pm and 8 pm. Most of the time my 2 pm meal is the largest meal of the day but often times it ends up being dinner with my husband at 6. My lightest meal of the day is the 8 pm meal because it's so late in the day. It's usually a piece of fruit, ¼ cup serving of nuts or a protein drink or smoothie. For you, however, I would recommend that from whatever time in the morning you start your first meal, plan to eat every three to four hours as best you can within the parameters of work, children, etc.

2.	Chose one meal a day to replace with a protein drink/shake or low sodium soup **(I have mine for breakfast at 8 am).**

3.	Choose a 150 to 200 calorie snack that you wouldn't mind eating up to two times a day. You can choose different types of snacks so that you can rotate for variety as long as it's under 200 calories or you may stick to the same thing every time **(I like to have a serving of fruit such as 10 grapes and 5 strawberries, or one Ataulfo mango or one Kiwi with 6 cubes of pineapple that** are 90 calories each WITH ½ Nature Valley Protein Chewy bar that's 95 calories usually at 11am and 8pm). I also like to have 12 tortilla chips and 1 TBSP of salsa, a small apple with 1 TBSP peanut butter or cocoa hazelnut spread, 5 Oreo® Thins or 2 fun size packages of Peanut M&M's®.

4.   Choose two meat and vegetable combinations that total no more than 500 to 600 calories each to use one for lunch and the other for dinner (**I usually have 4 oz. of meat (chicken, pork chop, stewed or roast beef, or tilapia) and a veggie (green beans, broccoli, spinach and greens) at 2pm (lunch) and meat (tuna or lean deli meat) and a salad around 6pm). Sometimes I choose poorly and I eat all my 1200 calories + one 180 calorie snack when I'm out for lunch, and I'm usually full for the rest of the day. But if I get hungry before bedtime I'll have a smoothie at 8. Lunch is my biggest meal. Most of the times I make the meat that we're going to have for dinner in time for my 2 pm meal and have it with a veggie or salad and I usually don't want it again for dinner; so I'll have a smoothie for dinner. Also if I have pasta for lunch, I'll have a smoothie for**

dinner (so that I can have as much pasta as I want for lunch.) See below for a look at what my eating plan looks like today. Please note that I worked my way down to this 1800 calories per day routine in 500 calorie increments. I also learned mindful eating and broke my addiction to sugar before I was strong enough to settle in to this plan. Remember, if I could do it, you can too. Also, only make the changes that you're comfortable making because it's only when you internalize that your choices are contrary to your goals that you can change in a way that keeps you from reverting back to old ways. If you try this and find out you have trouble sticking to it, continue with the quick 500, try the tea recipe and read further in the book for tools to resolve your food issues. Just keep finding ways to chip away at your caloric intake 500 calorie increments at a time. I know most people trying to lose weight should not eat late but that doesn't work for me because at least three nights of the week I am out in the evening. So I do need something after the usual dinner time, but it's very small and light. And it's protein and fruit.

MEAL	TIME	FOOD	CAL	
BRFST	**8 am**	**Protein drink**	**200**	
SNACK	**11 am**	**Fruit & ½ protein bar**	**200**	
LUNCH	**2 am**	**4 oz meat & veggie**	**620**	
DINNER	**6pm**	**4 oz meat & veggie**	**620**	
SNACK	**8pm**	**Fruit & ½ protein bar or smoothie**	**200**	

Total Calories   1840

Professor Haub Twist Journal

Feeling strong enough to slash more than 500 calories? Good. Write out your plan try to make you meals as close as possible to the amount in calories as listed.

Breakfast_(250cal)__________________________

____

Snack__(180cal)__________________________

____

Lunch__(400cal)__________________________

____

Snack__(180cal)__________________________

____

Dinner__(500cal)__________________________

____

Snack__(180cal)__________________________

____

____

Grocery List for Trena Tea

TEA BASE, Makes 2 quarts
Zest and juice of 2 lemons
1/4 pound ginger root
8 green tea bags (I use Lipton orange, passionfruit and jasmine flavored)
8 oz. organic apple cider vinegar (I use Bragg's)
8 oz. coconut water (pure and WITHOUT pulp—I use Vita Coco)
Pinch of baking soda
OILS
1 TBSP avocado oil or 1 TBSP extra virgin olive oil
1 TBSP coconut oil (Avoid any oil mixed with corn, vegetable, canola or animal oil.)

You may try a combination oil. Look for Carrington Farms avocado/coconut oil or for La Espanola avocado/olive oil

SPICES

3 Shakes of cayenne
3 Shakes of ground cinnamon
3 Shakes of ground turmeric

SWEETENERS (Optional)
2 TBSP honey
1 TBSP coconut palm sugar

Recipe for Tea Base

Cut ginger root into slices, place into a sauce pot, with 4 cups of water and bring to a boil. Put in 8 tea bags, cover with lid, turn off burner and allow the ginger and tea bags to sit in the steaming water so that the tea becomes infused with the ginger. Meanwhile, pour 8 oz. of vinegar, 8 oz. coconut water and the zest and juice of 2 lemons into a 2 quart container with a dispenser. After tea has brewed at least 15 minutes, pull out and discard the tea bags, pour tea along with the ginger slices from the sauce pot into the dispenser. Add water to dispenser to make 2 quarts. And that's the tea base.

How to Make a Serving from Tea Base

Pour 8 oz. of tea base into a cup. Add pinch of baking soda. Add 3 Shakes each of cinnamon, cayenne and turmeric. Add 1 TBSP each of the avocado oil and coconut oil. Use extra virgin olive oil if you do not have one of the others. Warm in microwave 1 minute. Sweeten to taste.

How to Make Tea by the Cup

Warm 8 oz. of water with 4 slices of ginger root in microwave 1 minute, put in 1 tea bag and allow to brew 2 minutes. Remove tea bag. Add lemon juice, 1 ounce of vinegar, 3 shakes of each spice and pinch of baking soda. Add 1 TBSP each of avocado and coconut oils. Warm 1 additional minute. Sweeten to taste.

Tips

TIGHT BUDGET— The average cost to buy everything in the recipe is $60 but if you'll make that initial investment; the non-perishable core items of the recipe will allow you to make the tea about three times. However, if you do not have the funds to cover the expenses for the entire recipe you may consider ordering Trena Tea online, then you'd only need to buy lemon, vinegar and oils to add to the brew, which should cost around $20. Oils get expensive plus it may be difficult to have 2 tablespoonful's worth in the tea so you may want to start by investing in one oil at a time or try a combination oil. If $20 is too much to spare right now, start by taking oils, which would cost about $8. I have found—La Espanola (Avocado/Olive Oil) or Carrington Farms (Avocado/Coconut Oil) are the most helpful but any of them will help you slim the belly. Try adding 1 TBSP in 4 oz. coffee, tea or warm coconut milk once daily. You'll be so pleased with the results that you may consider the complete recipe a worthy investment.

ALLERGIES— Please exclude any item from the recipe to which you have a known allergy.

RECOMMENDED FREQUENCY— Once daily. This is not a tea that you can guzzle down on the run, so drink it slowly to avoid choking. (If you truly need to take in the morning and drink it hurriedly, recommend decreasing or removing the cayenne. I have found the best time of the day is either in the morning on an empty stomach (so you have to set aside the time to sip it) or in the evening 1 hour before bedtime. For me I didn't see any different results beyond a one week's time frame. When in the process of losing weight, I would take the tea daily for 7 days to break any plateaus and help my body re-set to a lower weight. Since losing the weight, I maintain a flat belly by taking the tea once per week.

OILS --I began including oils in the tea because it takes **good fats** (monounsaturated, polyunsaturated and saturated) to burn fat and I was not using them enough in my meal plans so I put them in the tea. They are found in meats, nuts, butter, and cream.

SWEETENERS—Sweeteners are optional; use with caution. If you really want to avoid sweetener, put one half of the ginger in the tea boil. Then take the other half of the ginger and PEEL, GRATE and BLEND the ginger to a pulp. (*Then put the RAW, blended ginger into the dispenser along with the coconut water, apple cider vinegar and lemon juice.* Keeping everything else as per the recipe). It makes the tea have a rich, full and heady flavor. It will be cloudy at the bottom that's okay just stir it up before you serve it. I have found that when I take this extra step I do not need as much sweetener. Most of the time I'm moving too fast for the extra step and 2 TBSP of honey is enough and I do NOT need to use the coconut palm sugar at all. I've found that if we want the tea to help, we have to make it good to our own tastes so that we'll actually drink it. So it helps to add whole cinnamon sticks, the zest and juice of 2 oranges, a cup of tart cherries in the summer or a cup of cranberries in the fall to the tea and ginger brew in the sauce pan. If for some reason the tea doesn't taste pleasurable to me once it's in the cup, it helps to add an extra squeeze of lemon juice and/or a shake of ground ginger—(by the way ground ginger is best for the flavor factor only. There is not enough nutritional value in ground ginger to substitute for ginger root. And if adding lemon and ground ginger doesn't help, then I add an extra TBSP of honey. But if I happen to use distilled apple cider vinegar (which I've found to be more acerbic than the organic apple cider vinegar) or make my tea base too strong (which happens when I let it sit and brew so long that it becomes bitter) I dilute with water rather than adding sweetener.

STRAWS, LIDS AND STIRRERS-- I often use STIRRERS to stir the tea and sometimes sip the tea using a STRAW—again I can't stress enough-- slowly. The best tools I've found is to use disposable insulated CUPS WITH LIDS to assist with getting the oils down without them sticking to my lips or wreaking havoc on dishes. This makes it to where I can throw the cup away and the only dishware used is a tablespoon or a measuring spoon. Sometimes I just take the oils directly by mouth from a tablespoon so then I can sip on the tea and enjoy it without the oils floating around in there.

REFRIGERATION-- I do not bother to refrigerate the tea base because it has vinegar in it and should be gone in a week. If there is an amount that hasn't been used in a week I'll refrigerate it at that point. I DOUBLE THE RECIPE FOR TWO PEOPLE.

STICKY HONEY--I make sure to measure the oil before I measure the honey because then the honey doesn't stick to the spoon.

COMBINATION OILS-- Sometimes I find combination oils such as those listed in the grocery list which alleviates buying two or three different oils but then I'll use 2 TBSP of the combination oil. But you can decide if you can handle that much oil in your tea or not.

READ LABELS ON COCONUT WATER-- I AVOID using coconut water WITH PULP because I've found that they have more sugar and carbs (some as much as 45 grams per serving). So I check the label and make sure carbs/sugar is about 12 grams per 8 oz. serving.

THREE SHAKES-- Before I do the 3 shakes of the spices I bring the spice to the top of the lid of the container and then shake 3 times that way I get plenty of spice per shake. Make sure a good amount of spice comes out of the container each time you shake.

SKIN CARE—Take a couple dabs of either one of the oils and smooth on your face, neck, hands, arms and especially elbows.

AVOID TOXIC PEOPLE. STAY AWAY FROM PEOPLE WHO TRY TO PUT YOUR FIRE OUT. AVOID DREAM KILLERS.

Day of Reckoning

It was February of 2016, I seemed to not be able to lose more than 20 pounds and that 20 pounds I could never keep it off; so I had given up trying. The other thing that contributed to weight gain was that when I was finishing my undergraduate degree, four nights a week I ate out, due to lack of planning. Mondays and Wednesdays were church nights and Tuesdays and Thursdays were school nights. The day finally came when God arranged for me to stop ignoring this pink elephant in my life. It was time to pay up for my past mistakes. This was a test. Would I pass—figure out how to lose more than 20 pounds and keep it off; or fail—make no more effort to change and keep doing what I was doing? If there is something you need to do in life and you're not paying attention, life has a way of making you pay attention by putting up a brick wall that you can't get over, under, or around. You just have to go through. Somebody say, "Amen" for Life Interruptions!" I have found that the quicker you gain insight, the quicker the storm passes.

It was probably a very bad idea to set my appointment with my Endocrinologist so soon after vacation but it couldn't be delayed. My blood glucose levels averaged 180 every morning (not a good thing) after our trip to Orlando, Florida, so I had to go in. It was a wonderful trip, though! We stayed in the most luxurious suite ever at Sheraton Vistana Villas. It was a condo really—complete with kitchenette, living room, washer/dryer and it even had two televisions. We started off the week in Daytona Beach at NASCAR. Then at the Kennedy Space Center near Cape Canaveral we visited NASA's launch complex, observed various other types of space paraphernalia, perused the astronaut hall of fame. Then we experienced a simulated launch. We went to EPCOT (Experimental Prototype Community of Tomorrow) Center at Walt Disney World where we shopped, took the Chevrolet test drive and strolled around the boardwalk tasting food from around the world. At the Holy Land Experience we saw a replica of the Jerusalem temple, all our favorite bible story landmarks and experienced the most humorous, thought-provoking, exquisite performances that really brought the Bible to life. We caught a game between the Golden State Warriors and the Orlando Magic. All the while munching on decadent foods and rich desserts.

So it was no wonder that I found myself at the doctor's office because I couldn't get my blood sugar levels regulated. I expected my doctor to give me a hard time, not the bad news that he gave me. He prescribed an injection for me to take weekly and I immediately objected begging him to add on another pill. He looked at me above the top rims of his glasses and said, "Trena, Trena, Trena… You're already on three different medications." He told me he was constantly monitoring my organs closely because the medications were giving them a real good work out; that if this didn't bring my blood sugar under control, he'd have to put me on insulin. Then I'd have to deal with injections on a daily basis, several times a day, not just weekly. He told me that the weekly injections are said to help patients lose a few pounds. He suggested I use this long enough to get the sugar under control and possibly drop some weight to hopefully come off of the injections. He said with diet and exercise if I could lose about 40 pounds, I could be totally off all the medications. Here are the points he gave me:

Make eating right and exercise your medicine. Do this (take medications as prescribed) and then as soon as safe to do so (under doctor's care) make eating right and exercise my next "prescription" for keeping my blood sugar and high blood pressure under control.

Let go of the concept of quick, fast or effortless weight loss. A fad diet (a way of eating for a period of time until meeting a particular goal) to lose weight fast would not do. I should have a meal plan instead. This would require a lifestyle change with the occasional enjoyment of my favorite treats.

It's a battle. A major problem with weight loss is that the body doesn't understand that we're trying to reduce weight. **It's our body's job to MAINTAIN *THE WEIGHT THAT IT HAS*.** When the body senses that the caloric intake is less than 1/3 of what it usually receives and or activity increases, it slows metabolism to stop it. We call these plateaus. Knowing that they are a part of the process, makes it easier to build strategies to be ready for them. To overcome plateaus we have to mix up food and work out routines. This is all in an effort to sort of trick the body to reset, kick start the metabolism back into fat burning mode and accept a new, lower weight "norm" to maintain.

Slow and steady wins the weight-loss race. The biggest obstacle to losing the weight is that it is a slow process. The weight didn't get there overnight and it is not going to come off overnight; so be patient with the process. A nice slow weight loss minimum of at least 1 pound a week is sufficient progress.

One pound per week is a reasonable goal. In order to achieve fat loss, you need to burn more calories than you get from your food. That's called a caloric deficit. *A pound of fat contains around 3500 calories. So the logic is that if you create a DAILY caloric deficit of 500 calories over a 7-day period, that's equal to 3500 calories, which is 1 pound per week* (Walters, 2016). It's important to look at how what you do from day to day affects the changes in the body over a 7-day period.

Type II Diabetes is reversible. People all over the world get diseases for which there is no known cure, but Type II Diabetes is 100 % reversible with eating right and exercising.

I could only agree to the doctor's recommendation. But when I went to the pharmacy to pick up my prescriptions I was informed that my insurance didn't cover the injections and the cost was more than I could pay out of pocket. Also my insurance provider had updated its list of approved drugs so it no longer covered the Januvia or the Jardiance I was taking. I knew what was waiting for me if I went back to my doctor. I couldn't go forward temporarily taking a weekly injection to bring my sugar under control but neither could I go back to oral medications I had been taking. So it was either be on insulin which felt like a death sentence or lose the weight to reverse the diabetes. So was I to continue as I was or make the change?

The biggest thing I remember from my doctor was that I could reverse the diabetes and take the fitness approach towards a cure instead of taking the approach of treating the symptoms. **Also,** I'd seen it happen for family members so I hoped it would work for me.

My father, James, suffered from diabetes but he discovered that a huge part of his problem was fluid retention. He cut all sodium from his diet but was still retaining fluid. Then he and his doctor figured out that it was the 3 or 4 antacid tablets he was taking after almost every meal causing him to retain water. (which I took to mean 6 to 9 because most people take 2 or 3 tablets; up to three times per meal to get relief) So when he stopped taking those he lost 50 pounds and is doing a lot better. So I realized if my father could figure out what was causing him to hold onto his weight (even if it was mostly fluid), I could too.

Now my brother, Jimmy, found out he was diabetic. It scared him so badly-- knowing all the problems Dad was facing, he lost 60 pounds by avoiding sugar and carbohydrates and walking, walking, walking— A LOT meaning a whole bunch—with high intensity (getting his heart rate up to 135—he's 10 years younger than I am); and his blood sugar normalized.

The same happened for my grandmother, Bobbie Joyce Tennon. Even at an advanced age she went from a size 18W down to a size 14 (which was similar to my goal except I was a size 20W) by putting a stop to drinking syrupy sweet teas and lemonades that she had dearly loved; she stopped snacking by sticking to whole meals and began to take walks. She was no longer considered diabetic by the time she passed away due to other issues.

My pastor and his wife lost a lot of weight by walking in their neighborhood that's full of rolling hills. Every time we had a meal in the church's fellowship hall he would say things like, "I'm going to pass on the rice and bread and drink water instead of punch because I want a slice of that homemade pound cake." Those sort of things encouraged me to know that it was possible for me to be successful because I didn't have to totally deny myself everything but instead make good choices.

So if they could do it, I figured I could too. I needed to lose the weight or be on insulin. Was it time to pay the price for all the years of poor nutrition by doing the right things from now on or was I going to pay the ultimate price in favor of continuing with poor nutrition? I had a decision to make. Would I make the changes that I needed to make and mean it for real this time or would I assume the defeatist's position that making the changes would be too overwhelming to undertake and maintain for life?

I recalled what the doctor said about all the people in the world who have disease for which no cure has been found but for my disease I actually knew the cure. Going on insulin meant that the disease was winning but I'd have a better chance at winning with complete resolution if I fought inside-out (make lifestyle change) rather than outside-in (taking medication). I had the advantage of seeing family members successfully make the change by figuring out what was causing the weight gain; developing strategies to overcome their challenges and staying committed to the agreements they made to themselves.

The life preserver had been cast into the deep. I felt it was wrong for me to have the solution and still not want to participate in my own rescue mission. So this was it—my day of reckoning. This was a time that I'm being called to account for my actions. This was a time that I was being tested. I could no longer believe the falsehood that it was just too hard to lose the weight and keep it off because I'd seen people I know figure out what they needed to do and then they simply did it. No excuses. At 51 years of age I knew the choice I made here, would affect the quality of my senior years. What did I want these years over the hill to be like? Looking ahead, I knew that if I kept going as I was my daughter and my husband would be strapped with my care in possibly ten years. I had also seen family members lose their limbs, go blind, suffer heart disease and yes pass away. And I've known people that have had to be on dialysis. I certainly didn't want that to happen to me. Was I going to let myself drown or was I going to reach for the flotation device. Somebody say, "Amen" to the knowledge that a confused mind does nothing. But as soon as a decision is made it must be backed with immediate action. I chose life. I chose to lose the weight. I hope you choose life also.

Day of Reckoning Exercise

I am hoping that you will also make a fundamental decision today. You may not have realized that all the times you failed to do what you've needed to do for good health management you have been waving off the life boat. So let's make a firm, intentional decision about fitness today. We'll get into more details of what you're going to change next. For now I just want you to first MAKE THE DECISION on whether or not you are going ALL IN. And that doing the same ole' thing or NOT *figuring out what you need to do differently* is the same as CHOOSING to flag off the rescue.

So here's the question… ***ARE YOU GOING TO DO WHAT IT TAKES TO BE FIT *OR NOT*?** Please highlight or circle the choice that you're going to pattern the rest of your life on.

Highlight or circle your choice

I have chosen to keep doing what I've been doing and I'm NOT going to figure out what I need to do differently. I have chosen NOT to participate in my own rescue mission.

I have chosen to be committed to figuring out what changes I need to make; developing strategies to overcome my weight-loss challenges and keeping the agreements I make with myself to achieve those goals. I choose life.

Making the Decision to be Totally Committed Journal

I'm hoping in advance that you have chosen life. Jot down your thoughts and feelings regarding your choice for a new lifestyle. Change.

A One-Dimensional Approach to Weight Loss

There are many branches of fitness, and with this medical issue I was trying to figure out where I went wrong, so I didn't try to assimilate them all at once. And I believe that starting with a unidimensional approach that grew into a multi-dimensional approach contributed greatly to my success after numerous failed attempts at getting fit. Since, for me, eating right was a huge mass of confusion and I loved to eat the things that were SO bad for me SO much; I knew I couldn't keep any sort of food intake agreement for very long. I put aside attempting any sort of eating discipline—besides those two breakfast cuts I mentioned in the introduction I focused on getting myself moving. Having served in the Navy, I decided to focus on working out because it was the sector of fitness that I knew I could be committed to doing consistently for life. It was the least confusing, uncomplicated aspect for me to incorporate that also presented a minimal amount of resistance to my getting started. It was also a choice because I knew I'd receive success with any amount of increased activity being that I had been pretty much sedentary before. Then I made the agreement that when the weight stopped dropping 1 pound per week, I'd learn something new to layer on top of what was already in progress.

Without much ceremony I *JUST GOT STARTED*…using Leslie Sansone's DVD **Just Walk – Ultimate Five Day Walk Plan.** (Sansone, 2012) I went with her because that's what I had right there in the house. I didn't want to risk waiting until payday to go buy something more contemporary. Besides, it was never hard to talk myself into doing it since her workouts are not intimidating. I didn't have to be exact with the moves, I just had to walk. On this DVD she has five different 15 minute walks that each total a mile. Since I wanted to walk two miles per day, I could choose which two I wanted to do daily to have some variation. On the weekend I could do all five and walk five miles! Then I would use the toning exercises she included to focus on certain areas. I also use a more up-to-date one called **Walk Off Fat Fast; Fat Burning Walks**

(Sansone L. , 2014) that doesn't focus so much on how many miles are completed but on fat burning intensity. There are 20 minute, 30 minute or 40 minute workouts. The other DVD I love is Jillian Michaels **Beginner Shred** (Michaels, 2014). She offers three 20-minute workouts that are to be used 10 days each. So in a 30 day period you get some really good results. I wouldn't describe this workout as fun, but it was, and is, oh so worth it. I keep going back to it because it keeps me losing the inches in all the places I want to shrink. Getting positive results from working out was extremely motivating because it set me on a path of getting my body to look the way I want it to look. As long as I was losing at least one pound per week I didn't sweat the fact that I wasn't doing *everything possible all at the same time* to reach my eventual goal.

Working out first really worked for me. And because my goal was to lower my blood sugar, I quickly learned that working out daily was the best frequency for me. So I really had to work hard to develop ways to make working out a priority EVERY DAY to avoid falling back into vegging out on the sofa. So not only did I start moving but I found ways to make it a DAILY part of my life as a new habit.

One-Dimensional Approach to Fitness Exercise

I got started by working out. Now it's time for you to decide what branch of fitness you can start *today* as a lifestyle change.

Items to start— Choose an exercise that burns 250 to 500 more intentional calories per day; practice mindful eating; practice nutritional eating (eating foods with nutritional value, rather than empty calories); drink sufficient water; use tea recipe for 7 days as a way to jump start metabolism; find support group,; subscribe to Perfect Meal Plans.com or a service like Hello Fresh®, for food prep and recipe ideas. Consider a system like Weight Watchers, Jenny Craig, Nutri-System with the understanding that you'll still have to transition from their foods to every day food; consider a weight loss clinic or nutritionist; join a gym or fitness center that includes a specialist to assist with generating a plan in reaching goals; get a personal trainer; try cardio, resistance training, high intensity interval training and or weight training videos and rotate them to give your body variation of movement; download My Fitness Pal.com application as a food journal; buy an activity tracker   like Fitbit.____

____

____

____

Items to stop—wean self off soda, limit bread that is not whole grain and chips, practice abstinence in regards to junk food (most fast foods, anything processed & fried), lattes, sugary drinks, and sweets.

____

____

____

____

Items to change—for favorite foods/drinks that you don't plan to give up decide how they are going to fit in your new meal plan.

Can you do a smaller size? Decide the frequency that you will allow yourself to have the treat. Can you substitute?

____

____

____

____

____

____

If already started a program and have hit a plateau, decide what you are going to do differently to get your metabolism going again. I highly recommend *Shred: The Revolutionary Diet* by Dr. Ian Smith. He gives an eating an exercise plan that you repeat in 6 week cycles until you meet your goal. And it changed everything for me. Also, try high intensity interval training, kettlebell, burpees or weight training. An infusion of consistent exercise will best help your body find its center, but it's a good idea to review your food journal for ways to go leaner. Weight loss is 80% nutrition and 20% work out. Make sure eating a sufficient amount of calories—especially protein and good fats, daily to support your activity. Sometimes people take their calorie count too low and stall their own plan. Sometimes others need to change their eating plan if they eat the same things all the time. Try Trena tea 7 days. Try reducing alcoholic beverages. Drink plenty of water.

____

____

____

____

Build Strategies to make it stick. Think about obstacles that keep you from staying committed to programs that work. Plan strategies to overcome those obstacles. For example, you find that you get busy making dinner, taking care of family and cleaning in the evenings. So you put a stationary bike and workout gear in the garage so you can pull into the garage, change and work out before you even go into the house.

____

____

Mindful Eating

Cutting 500 calories and working out worked for two weeks, but when I weighed myself at the beginning of the third week, I'd hit a plateau. I conceded that it was time to get started on eating right to take me to the next level. I still wasn't ready to totally give up eating all the foods I loved at that point so I focused on mindful eating. Mindful eating is the practice of deliberately taking note of every sensory experience associated with eating. It re-wires the brain and restores intuitive wisdom around eating. It helps break overeating and snacking; and helps to establish sustainable habits. (Lockhart, 2014) This is where the importance of a support group, physician or weight-loss program comes into play because a support group is where I got the concept from. Additionally, I learned the following very important tips from the Sports and Health Ministry at my church, Philadelphia Missionary Baptist Church, Kirby, Texas (near San Antonio):

Wait for hunger. Eat only when hungry. Fix your mind with the understanding that if you're not hungry, you shouldn't eat. At this point I still didn't concentrate on what I ate, I focused on *waiting* for hunger and *choosing* what to eat. So if I wanted a Snickers® bar, I could have it. But I had to wait for the stomach rumble before I could eat it and then not eat again until I was hungry again. I know some fellow church members who found themselves not eating full meals—sort of nibbling all day, trying to eat in this manner and I found myself doing the same thing. I did better when I had a planned meal or a snack prepared ahead of time for when hunger strikes arrived. So this is a good tool if you were like me… I didn't have to be hungry to eat. I would often get a taste for something and that would drive me to go get it and eat it. However, waiting for hunger helped me to stop a lot of in-between-meal snacking and choosing what to eat helped me stop grazing on auto-pilot.

Eat slowly, stop when full. Slow down so you can stop when you're satisfied to avoid overeating. It takes 20 minutes for your stomach to let your brain know that it's full. (Steen, 2016) Sit down at a table for your meals. Put fork down or sit back in the chair between bites. Start with eating the meat or most favorite food that's on your plate. Chew your food thoroughly. Chew slowly so that it's easier to recognize fullness. Stop when satisfied because if you feel stuffed, you've gone past full. So eat only when you're hungry and chew slowly so you can stop when you're full.

Make sure there's something on your plate that you enjoy. I have found that if you do not get a pleasure lift from your meal, you only end up with a hankering for something more after you've just had a full meal. Then you totally blow your meal plan, not because you didn't get enough in your nutritional meal but because you didn't get the pleasure kick from that meal.

Sweet water. One of the things I learned from the support group was that the body could go through some tremendous withdrawal symptoms and they recommended what I call sugar water to help cope with the changes that can occur with waiting. Put 4 oz. of orange juice (or juice of any flavor) in 32 oz. of water and sip on it throughout the day to combat cravings and crankiness that can come with waiting for hunger.

Learning to wait for hunger was crucial to my fitness evolution because if I didn't feel hunger pains but felt an urge to eat, the cause was likely boredom or stress or as Dr. Phil explains in his book, **The Ultimate Weight Solution: The 7 Keys to Weight Loss Freedom** (McGraw, 2003) it meant that I was "sad, mad or glad." So if there's no stomach rumble yet there's a desire to eat it's best to ask yourself what's going on that you're using food to feel better. You need to analyze your food journal and look for any patterns and seek to find out when the need to eat out of turn strikes. Then come up with strategies and alternatives. If not hungry you need to find other methods to cope with being stressed, mad or sad rather than using food to self-medicate. For boredom and gladness, we need to seek non-food related ways to fill time or to celebrate. Learning when to eat by waiting for body signals and having the awareness to stop when full is a dimension of fitness that is often overlooked.

Mindful Eating Exercise

Try mindful eating with the twist that I applied.
1. Once you eat your first meal of the day (not whatever you want as the system prescribes, but what you have planned) then plan to eat every 3 to 4 hours. If you plan and prep your meals you won't have to worry so much about portions because you've already weighed and measured out the food. **If you feel an urge to eat but you're not physically hungry, that's when you self-coach, "Nope, going to wait for hunger or my next planned meal time." You may consider taking a brief walk or having a 100 calorie snack to get you past the moment if you're really distressed. I often have a tea, a mint, chew gum or have a pack of smoky almonds. Check to see if you have a taste in your mouth, because you might just need to drink warm water.**
2. To keep from snacking and eating out of turn remember to **WAIT FOR HUNGER**, *SAVOR EACH MEAL* and **EAT SLOWLY** so that you'll be better able to *STOP WHEN FULL*.

Mindful Eating Journal

Jot down your experiences regarding Mindful Eating. For example, how do you feel sitting down to eat rather than standing at your kitchen counter?

____

____

____

____

____

____

____

____

____

____

____

____

.Know Your Chemistry

While mindful eating is a dimension of fitness that is often overlooked, the other one is individualized chemistry. In this chapter, I'm going to layer on additional information to go with the "Quick 500" exercise provided in the introductory chapter regarding intake versus caloric expenditure to get you to another level. Also I will share a list of fitness facets I'd been overlooking regarding the chemistry of eating and exercise that turned out to be extremely important in my journey that I think will be very helpful to you if you apply sooner rather than later:

We are the weight that we are because we EAT calories more consistently than we BURN calories. Our goal here is to change that around. So after you determine where you are, I'll give you the formula to take steps to change it. Also I will include tools to help you be more exact in knowing how many calories you are truly burning as you do your intentional activities; then follow up with the list fitness facets.

First, you need to know where you are. This is the rate at which your body burns calories at rest—basal metabolic rate (BMR) or resting metabolic rate (RMR). This is the amount of calories required to maintain your current weight. To calculate it out manually take your current weight and multiply by 12 (activity level). (**Note**: Use 12, if almost never exercise, 13.5 for moderate exercise for 3 to 5 days a week and 15.5 for vigorous exercise 6 to 7 days a week) (Solo, 2014). There is also a calculator available on the website of the American Council of Exercise that will provide a general caloric goal to prevent weight gain. The web address is www.acefitness.org; click Tools for Life; click Tools & Calculators; click Daily Caloric Needs Estimate Calculator. Enter your age, weight, sex, height in feet and inches and select activity level. The answer the calculator gives is how many calories you should eat each day to maintain the weight you are (American Council of Exercise, 2017).**This tells us where you are.** The amount of calories you're currently taking in and your current level of activity is what's keeping you at the weight that you are now. If you have a food journal pick a 7 day period. Add the total calories for the week and divide by 7 to calculate the average. Your seven day average should come in at close to your BMR. The amount in the calculator will be slightly higher than your average so that you avoid gaining weight.

Second, you need to know how to alter your current state to lose the weight. Increase physical activity to burn an intentional 500 calories per day or reduce food intake 500 calories per day or do a combination of exercise increase to burn 250 and decreased food intake of 250 that total at least a 500 to caloric deficit. So in my case I weighed 250 pounds and was pretty sedentary. So 250 x 12 = 3000 for my BMR. Which is about right to explain where I was at the start of my program because I used to consume around 3000 calories a day. I began by changing breakfast to create a 500 calorie deficit and began working out which was about a 300 calorie burn.(Which was more than the 500 calorie minimum, so gave me wiggle room)

Calories Burned
In normal day 3000 + Just Walk 300 = 3300
VS.
Calories Eaten 3000 – 500 (Swapped coffee for frappe and 1 taco instead of two) = 2500
Shows a 800 calorie deficit

So the changes worked because I was able to create a deficit with **consistency**. Recall that it's a matter of chemistry. **One pound of fat is equal to 3500 calories.**

Remember that creating at least a 500 calorie deficit PER DAY for a 7 DAY PERIOD equals 3500 calories which yields a loss of 1 pound of FAT per week.

Take a look at this example that can give you an idea of how you can perhaps miss the mark. Let's say that you currently use 1800 calories a day to maintain current weight (BMR) but you actually eat 2300 calories. Although you track 10,000 steps (with enough intensity to burn 500 calories) you'd have no change in weight loss because you haven't created a deficit (Walters, 2016).

Calories Burned
In normal day 1800 + 10,000 Steps 500 = 2300
VS.
Calories Eaten = 2300

However if you stick to your eating plan and consumed 1800 calories a day (BMR) and you track 10,000 steps, you'd create a deficit in your favor for weight loss.

Calories Burned
In normal day 1800 + 10,000 Steps 500 = 2300
VS.
Calories eaten = 1800

Go beyond. Now, if you feel that you are strong enough to go to the next level instead of a 500 calorie deficit, you'll want to know how to do it without cutting your calories so low that you go into starvation mode. You get there by reducing your calorie intake by a third of your current BMR. Here's the formula:

(Weight X Activity level), which is your BMR and $\div$ 3 = which is maximum amount of calorie deficit (1/3 of your BMR) (. Now subtract this amount from BMR and this is your new calorie intake goal.

Note: Use 12, if almost never exercise, 13.5 for moderate exercise for 3 to 5 days a week and 15.5 for vigorous exercise 6 to 7 days a week (Solo, 2014)

Try it again.

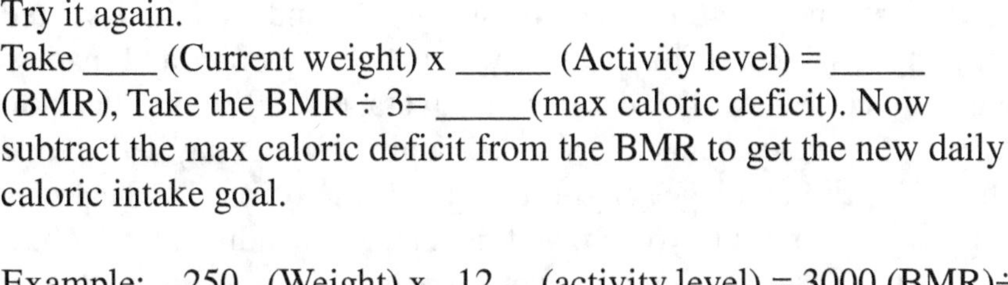

Take _____ (Current weight) x ______ (Activity level) = ______ (BMR), Take the BMR ÷ 3= ______(max caloric deficit). Now subtract the max caloric deficit from the BMR to get the new daily caloric intake goal.

Example:__250_ (Weight) x _12__ (activity level) = 3000 (BMR)÷ 3= 1000. So then 3000 (BMR) – 1000 = 2000 calories per day

So you may recall that I'd changed my breakfast, started working out and began mindful eating but those changes brought me to an 800 calorie deficit that only took me so far. So that's when I decided on adjusting my snacks by getting a variety box of 100 calorie snacks to eat instead of chips and candy and instead of sweet tea, I changed to water (So making changes to two snack meals brought my second 500 calorie deficit).

Changed Breakfast
Calories Burned
In normal day 3000 + Just Walk 300 = 3300
VS.
Calories Eaten 3000 – 500 (Swapped coffee for frappe and 1 taco instead of two) = 2500
Shows a 800 calorie deficit

Changed snacks/ Changed activities
Calories Burned
In normal day 2500(BMR) + Just Walk DVD 300 + 5000 steps 200= 3000
VS.
Calories Eaten 2500 – 500 Changed to 100 calorie snacks and water) = 2000
Shows a 1000 calorie deficit

After I stopped getting results with the second deficit, I started bringing my lunch (This change was my third deficit and made a huge impact because I went from an average 1300 calorie lunch to a 500 - 600 calorie lunch.) I kept dropping by making better food choices until I could get myself to a point where I ate 1840 calories per day. So hopefully you are getting an understanding that it's best to work your way towards your goal in increments that you personally set. *It's like a fat-burning bonfire in which you decide what you're going to contribute to keep the fire going.*

So you can use this formula to track your physical activity against your food intake over a seven day period to better enable you to determine where you may be falling short; and you can know if you truly need to stick to your meal plan and/or fitness regimen or have room to relax it a little.

Third, know the metabolic value of your exercise. Physical Activity Calorie Counter/MET Minutes
The metabolic equivalent of task (MET), or metabolic equivalent is the physiological measure expressing the energy cost (calories) of physical activities. It is the ratio of the rate of energy expended during an activity TO the rate of energy expended at rest. So MET value indicates the intensity of an activity compared to being at rest. (Ainsworth BE, 2011)For example, watching television or sitting at rest has a MET of 1.0 and an activity, like bicycling greater than 10 mph, that has a MET of 5. So the activity is five times the number of calories as sitting at rest.

A MET minute is the time engaged in the activity times the equivalent of task. So 30 minutes engaged in MET of 5 would be 150 MET minutes. (Hughes, 2012) The American Council for Exercise also as a calculator for that. Go to acefitness.org. Click on Tools for Life, then Tools & Calculators then click on Physical Activity Calorie Counter. You'd need to enter weight and hours spent. Then select activity and it will provide a number for calories burned. *The frequency, intensity and duration of a person's workout all contribute to calories burned through physical activity.*

Health Indicators

Body Mass Index (BMI) is a convenient way to estimate how much fat is on your body. Your BMI is a good number to know because it can help you determine your risk for dangerous health conditions associated with increased body fat. As being overweight or obese means you are at higher risk for premature death.

Calculate your BMI number by entering your height and weight into the BMI Calculator at American Council of Exercise.org. Go to Tools for Life; click Tools & Calculators; click BMI Calculator. Then find your BMI category on the following table to determine if you're underweight, normal weight, overweight or obese. (American Council of Exercise, 2017)

BMI Number	BMI Range
18.5	Underweight
18.5 -24.9	Normal weight
25 – 29.9	Overweight
30 – 34.9	Grade I Obesity
35- 39.99	Grade II Obesity
>40	Grade III Obesity

There are differences in opinion in regards to the use of BMI because it does not take into account that muscle weighs more than fat, so then a muscular person's numbers may put them in an obese or overweight range that is not accurate. A muscular person may want to consider using Waist Circumference.

Waist Circumference

Measure your waist anchoring the measuring tape 1 inch above your belly button. A woman whose waist circumference is greater than 35 inches (86 cm) or man whose circumference is greater than

40 inches (102cm) are at high risk of high blood pressure, heart attack, stroke, Type 2 Diabetes, breathing problems and certain cancers.

Body composition and size matters. Note that high intensity interval training and weight training have the benefit of continuing the fat burning up to 24 hours *after* the work out—depending on the intensity. Also, note that what most affects your basal metabolic rate (BMR), the rate at which your body burns calories at rest, is body composition and size. In regards to composition, a pound of muscle burns 14 calories whereas a pound of fat burns up to 3 calories per day (Solo, 2014) So try to gain muscle as quickly as you can. In regards to size, a heavier person uses more energy to move than a lighter person. (Walters, 2016)

I found this table (see below) on an information website regarding a walk from NJ to NY that may better help you understand the differences between weight and distance walked against speed (intensity). Note that the numbers across the top are intended to mean the participants' weight. The numbers inside the box are calories burned. Also note the following breakdown of the speeds 2 mph is casual pace, 3 mph is moderate pace, 4 mph is a very brisk pace, and 5 mph is very fast pace. There are some good calculators out there but I have found this formula to work for me:

Your Weight _______ X Distance_________ = Energy Used (Calories burned) Walking

Calories Burned Per Mile by Walking

Speed	150lb	160lb	180lb	200lb	220lb
2mph	85.5	91	102	114	120
3mph	79.5	85	95	106	112
4mph	85.5	91	102	114	120
5mph	109	116	131	145	160

The article gives the following note about the above chart, "You burn more calories per miles at very low speeds because you are basically starting and stopping with each step and your momentum isn't helping to carry you along. Meanwhile at very high walking speeds you are using more muscle groups with arm motion and with race-walking stride. Those extra muscles burn up extra calories with each step." (Kiczek, 2017)

Have a doctor's visit. See your doctor to check hormone and cholesterol levels. Check for vitamin and mineral deficiency that you may need to take supplements for. You may find that you have a thyroid condition. Also check hydration level, you may even find out that the many times you felt an urge to eat, your body was really craving water.

Drink plenty of water. Instead of taking sips recommend that you take 5 swallows (½ cup) to 10 swallows (1 cup) at a time because your body can do more with those quantities than little drops. Besides plain water there's Acidic water that helps with digestion and belly fat. If not on the tea, I drink acidic water—2 tbsp. of apple cider vinegar in a cup of water, on an empty stomach in the mornings. There's also Alkaline water, which is purified, oxygenated water infused with select minerals that help with body aches and makes one feel rejuvenated, alive and perky all over. I try to drink 6 to 8 glasses of water daily and most of the time it's alkaline water. I use Viva H20. It has phosphates and electrolytes to help with hydration. There are also mixes that you can pour into bottled water to add electrolytes that help you hydrate, just check the label to watch for those with a lot of sodium or sugars.

Diet book that helped the most. I highly recommend *Shred: The Revolutionary Diet* by Dr. Ian Smith, M.D. (Smith, 2012) He gives an eating and exercise plan that you repeat in 6 week cycles until you meet your goal. I like it because the foods he prescribes are on your grocery list any way. It's remarkable easy to follow. You do the first 6 weeks exactly he states but if you need additional cycles to meet your goal you choose which order you want to do them. There's lot's of flexibility to switch things up and make it your own and over 200 recipes.

Disordered food behavior. If you feel the urge to eat but your stomach hasn't grumbled you're experiencing disordered eating behavior. ***Food is to be used as fuel to the body and you should only fill up when the tank is empty.*** So take the time to figure out what is driving you to eat out of order. It's usually some sort of stress for which you need to find some other method of coping than eating. To avoid emotional eating develop strategies such as taking a brief walk, repeating a mantra like "Wait for the hunger" or choosing a pre-determined "go - to" snack to eat that will get you passed the urge but doesn't wreck your eating plan. Again, I say, sometimes an urge to eat is often times an urge to drink water because we either drink something other than water when thirsty or ignore thirst signals altogether.

Frequency of eating. Although you're waiting for hunger, plan to eat every 3 to 4 hours, unless you've eaten a heavy meal. ***A direct result of undereating is overeating***.

Plan what to eat. Not only should you plan when to eat, you should plan what you're going to eat daily on a morning empty stomach, breakfast, AM snack, lunch, PM snack, dinner and evening empty stomach. Once you have determined what you're going to eat, prepare it ahead of time so that it's readily available just like fast food.

Work scheduled eating. If you work in an environment where your eating is scheduled—then you can't afford to use 20 minutes of a 30 minute lunch time to figure out when you're full, so portion control is going to be important for you. Only prepare what you know will fill you up.

Note from the peanut gallery. If you've been doing this kind of work that doesn't allow more than 30 minutes for lunch and you've been there for more than a year you need to figure out what you need to do to get promoted-- unless this is all you *want* to do and the income provided is sufficient for your needs. Why do I say one year because in this day and age I have learned that when you start working for a place where you want more, you should be so impressive that within a year's time they are moving you up. That's right, if you're a call center representative you need to figure out what your company wants to hear on every call and wow them on every scale of measurement that they have until they move you up. A bad manager is inconsequential because competence is irrefutable. Don't worry about a manager that is trying to keep you pigeon-holed because your promotion can come from a level above frontline management. All the *manager's* boss (director) does is look at reports. You're going to have your name at the top of all of them. You need to be at least the top five of every standard of measurement and far exceeding in a few to where your boss's boss wants to know who you are and why you're in the same place. The higher up the ladder you go, the better you can control your schedule and improve your health. ***The more satisfied you are with life, the less you have a need to placate yourself with food.***

Journal what you eat. It will help you keep track, watch for patterns and analyze where you can make changes. I use My Fitness Pal.com.

Handling danger zones. Know your danger zones. It is extremely important to sit down and identify the intersections where the new habits need to replace the bad habits. So that you'll know to shore yourself up when you're in a spot that's full of temptation. Then plan tactics to get past the danger zone without wrecking yourself. You may want to start with these two: shopping and eating. **For shopping**, every time you get ready to go into a store review your commitment. Agree on a budget, what you are going to buy and what you are NOT going to buy. Put your commitment agreement in your phone where you can easily access it for review. Every store, even a hardware store has goodies. You know where the goodies are in the store so avoid those aisles. If you're going grocery shopping try going to a store like Whole Foods until you gain some control because they do not have candy, chips and soda around the register when you're trying to check out. **For eating**, if you planned your meals and then prepared them ahead of time so that they're readily available then you're not put in the position of having to decide what you're going to eat on the spur of the moment. But if you do, don't eat on autopilot. Decide what you're going to eat. Own it. Before buying food or putting food in your mouth, put the following questions in your phone and ask yourself, "Am I stomach-rumble hungry? If not, can I get by with peppermint, chew gum or a have a snack like a 100 calorie pack of Blue Diamond Smokehouse Almonds? Am I on autopilot or choosing this meal? What is the nutritional value of what I'm going to eat? Is this a food item on that's a part of my meal plan? If not healthy, can I substitute, eat half now and other half next day? Can I have a smaller size or share with someone else?"

If at a fast food restaurant and cannot get a salad, or do not _want_ a salad, have a kid's meal.
You can't outrun your fork. There's no amount of exercise that can cancel out a diet full of processed foods, junk foods and liquid calories. For example, a Big Mac, large fry and a large drink is 1350 calories, you'd have to walk 13.5 miles (To burn 100 calories per mile-- or 8.5 miles to burn off 850 extra calories (1350 – 500 amount of calories in a healthy meal) to zero it out. You can have the meal but you'll want to plan how you're going to increase your exercise or cut back on future meals so that the treat doesn't derail your fitness goals. What you eat is responsible for 70 to 80 per cent of weight-loss success. (Freedhoff, 2014) The focus should be on forming new eating habits.

Weigh in weekly rather than daily. I discovered that when I'd _gained_ weight on a daily weight check I found myself discouraged, even depressed and apt to cheat. And even when I _lost_ weight on a daily weight check I was _still_ apt to cheat because I would tell myself that I was doing so well that it was okay to lighten up. I found myself on a weight-loss defeating, emotional roller coaster all for naught. Three to four pound daily weight gain fluctuations are often caused by hormones, dehydration, sodium intake and various other body functions; not real fat gain. Weighing in weekly provided the impetus to choose wisely from day to day for fear of going a whole week and having little or no progress.

Be kind to yourself. I learned to be gentle and patient with myself realizing that this is a process and the journey was just as important as the destination. I learned to reframe "failures" as "setbacks" to use as learning experiences rather than self-deprecating tactics.

One slip up does not have to ruin the whole day. I learned that it was important to be present while eating so that I could enjoy *all* foods whether it was quinoa and kale or cake and ice cream. I no longer engage in all-or-nothing; good or bad thinking about foods because that is also disordered eating behavior. So if I eat a cherry-filled donut for breakfast I give myself permission to do so for that one meal. It means that I've used my carb allowance for the day on the donut and will stick to lean proteins and veggies for the rest of the day or add a little more intensity at workout time. It doesn't have to lead to an entire day of fattening foods. This helped stop the pendulum swinging between deprivation and bingeing

Get physical. I think exercise should be done daily. Exercise doesn't have to be boring or make you miserable. It should be 20 to 45 minutes—no longer than an hour, of an activity that elevates the heart rate and takes the body outside of its normal comfort zone.

Make it fun. Choose a physical activity that you enjoy doing for FUN that doesn't feel like a workout routine and do it weekly or a couple of times per month. Like visiting the national parks in your area and enjoying biking or hiking. Try visiting the latest exhibit in town but wear comfortable shoes and walk the whole museum. Try dancing, swimming, rock climbing or martial arts. For example, gardening can burn 200 to 400 calories per hour.

Get plenty of rest. Before you go to bed you need to unplug to get a good night's sleep. I turn off my television, phone and computer. I do my workout. I bathe or shower. I take whatever I've planned to have on my PM empty stomach. Then I read scripture, pray, meditate then concentrate on silence so that I can sleep well.

Be prepared for plateaus. Regarding meals, once you rid yourself of junk food, sweets and fast food begin a meal plan that includes protien, meats and fish; good oils found in meats, avocado, quinoa, nuts and seeds; fiber like lintels and black beans. If you get to a point to where you're eating right, but still hit a plateau, go from having a lean menu with no more than 30grms of carbs per day to having a treat day (some people call these cheat days) where you would be allotted more carbs, 50 grams (sweet potatoes, quinoa, and pasta, pizza) on that day but then eat lean the rest of the week. This variation or "confusion", along with the tea recipe will help break through the plateau and turn the fat burning back on. **Regarding exercise**, you should do as many full body exercises as possible. Try weight training. I like Kelly Coffey-Meyer, **30 Minutes to Fitness—Muscle Up Lift 2B Fit**. You may also want to include resistance training and High Intensity Interval Training (HIIT).   High Intensity Interval Training is creating exercise with intensity that generates a breathlessness (oxygen debt) alternating with periods of rests. The oxygen debt creates the atmosphere to where your body burns fat in anticipation that you will need more energy. Whereas with moderate exercise your body may use sugar in the blood first. So intensity encourages your body to burn fat. HIIT, resistance training (with bands or using body weight such as squats, lunges, planks and jumping jacks; and weight training not only help burn fat while working out but they create what's called after burn—for the next 24 to 48 hours after the exercise, muscles are still burning fat. That's why it's important to alternate weight training and HIIT with cardio. So you'd have a weight day; then a cardio day; a HIIT day and another cardio day. I like Cathe Friedrich's DVD **Ripped with HIIT: Low Impact HIIT** because she presents a low impact HIIT that easy on the knees and the back. I also enjoy the ten minute HIIT Butt Lift routine by Christine Bullock on **The 10 Minute Solution Butt Lift** DVD. There are times when I do not feel like following a DVD so then what I will do is get on my elliptical bike for 20 to 30 minutes alternating between a low, casual pace for a 1 minute interval with a high intensity fast pace in 3 minute intervals.

Know Your Chemistry Exercise

Know your BMR: _____ (Weight) x ______ (activity level) = ______ (BMR)

Weight _________ X 12 is the amount of calories to maintain the weight that you are.

Note: Use 12, if almost never exercise, 13.5 for moderate exercise for 3 to 5 days a week and 15.5 for vigorous exercise 6 to 7 days a week

Set a goal to go beyond a 500 calorie deficit to cutting back a THIRD of BMR
_____ (Weight) x ______ (activity level) = ______ (BMR) ÷ 3= _____max deficit, Then subtract max deficit from BMR.

Example: Let's say you weigh 180 pounds, take 180 x 12 = 2160 (BMR) ÷ 3= 720.
So 2160 (BMR) -720 = 1440 is amount you want to reduce caloric intake to.

Know your BMI. __________ Weight ÷ _________ height Use the table within the chapter to determine whether or not you have a health risk.

Try the Physical Activity Calorie Counter that is located at acefitness.com (Details on how to find the Fit for Life Tools are in the chapter) so that you can know how many calories are burned during different types of activities performed. Then choose two or three different ones that you like that will create the deficit you need and are willing to make the time to complete. This way you can rotate your work routines and not get bored.

Work your way, to where your meal plan is 1/3 of your BMR and you exercise an intentional 500 calories per day.

Search You Tube for cardio, Zumba, yoga, Pilates, weight training and High Intensity Interval Training DVD's to see the different exercises out there so that you can decide which ones you want to invest in and get started doing. I like Jillian Michaels, Cathe Friedrich, Kelley Coffey-Meyer and Christine Bullock. Remember that it's best not to do HIIT and Weight Training every day or you'll make that rookie mistake of making yourself sick. You must rotate HIIT- Cardio-Weight Training- Cardio- HIIT- Cardio-Weight Training- Cardio

Know Your Chemistry Journal

       Log your thoughts regarding weight-loss chemistry. What did you already know? Were you actually putting into practice the things that you knew? What was new information for you? Did any of the information lead to a motivation to start doing somethings differently? Write your experiences? Do you suddenly find that you have more will power and control knowing what you know now?

____

____

____

____

____

____

____

____

____

____

____

So Sick of Eating I Didn't Know What to Do

So I began with exercise then I layered on the dimension of mindful eating. I was able to continue losing, still slowly (because my meals were still primarily fast foods) but steadily. Fortunately for me about the same time that I hit the next plateau I saw on a local variety afternoon news show, *S.A. Live,* a segment about cold laser fat sculpting. They offered a 50% discount for the first 20 callers so I called and made an appointment. The program was explained to me. The Zerona laser makes little tears in fat cells so that fat cells break down and the body excretes the fat as normal. Mostly I wanted to get rid of my belly fat so I agreed to an 8 week plan and paid. I went back the next week for blood work and an assessment and was pleased that I'd dropped from 245 pounds to 230 pounds on my own in 6 weeks that had passed. Going into week seven I started this program.

Week(s)	Progress	Strategy
1	4lbs	Just Walk DVD
2	4lbs	Cut 500 +Just Walk DVD
3	No progress	So added Mindful Eating
4	4lbs.	Cut 1000 + DVD + Mindful Eating
5	3 lbs.	Cut 1000 + DVD + Mindful Eating
6	No progress	So found clinic

What is significant to note is that if I'd started exercising *and* eating right at the same time from the beginning I estimate that after the first 3 weeks I would have felt stalled early on with very little that I could change to continue increasing metabolism momentum. However by starting with one small change (exercise) adding another after each stall I had progress for a longer length of time (six weeks) which was a more gratifying, positive experience—and I had yet another dimension (eating the *right* foods for lunch and dinner) that I could layer on to take me further. I'd lost 15 pounds in 6 weeks without feeling tortured. So this is how the progression went, which is also the order of this book. I started with the one-dimensional approach of low impact exercising which worked for two weeks. Then layered on learning how to eat properly which helped another two weeks then went to the fat sculpting clinic where I learned that I wasn't eating enough of the right foods and until I got used to it I was so sick of eating I didn't know what to do. The fat sculpting was an eight week program focused on my outside but four weeks into the program I hit a plateau so I had to work on the inside which meant I had to break the chains of my addiction to refined sugar and starches. Forming a meal planning strategy for post fat sculpting I learned about healthy oils found in fish, lean meats, avocados, olives, nuts and seeds; anti-inflammatory and anti-oxidant properties of lemons, apple cider vinegar and coconut water, ginger, cinnamon, turmeric and cayenne. I wasn't including them in my cooking and learned about smoothies as a way to include them. I didn't like the way the ingredients tasted in smoothies but the earthy flavor of those ingredients reminded me of way tea tastes. So I decided to put them in a tea to get the nutrients in and – eureka! I've been able to maintain by staying away from dream killers, developing mental strength and exercising my faith. And finally I was onto a new beginning and I hope you begin yours as well.

So the third phase of my journey was working with the fat sculpting clinic. Once I met the doctor there, I was informed that for this program to be effective I couldn't expect to melt fat and continue to eat fat. So under the doctor's care I was put on a diet of 800 calories per day.

Warning:
Please do NOT attempt an 800 calorie per day diet without being under doctor's care because you will only harm yourself. For this plan to work *I had to take three different*

types of oral supplements, appetite suppressants, hormone injections, as well as vitamin injections. (Funny how I didn't want to be on insulin because of the injections but I agreed to do this—mainly because it was temporary). *All of the medication I had to take required prescriptions. So a low calorie diet like this one is not something you can do from home on your own safely without medical supervision.*

So, they explained the 800 calorie per day plan. For exercise I could walk if I wanted to but it was explained to me that I was not eating enough to do more than 30 minutes of light exercise—like walking, three times a week. On the days for walking I could add 200 calories of protein per day. "800 calories per day? Seriously?" was my response. She told me that ***I probably consumed about 3000 calories per day but because most of it was junk food my body could only use about 500 of the 3000 calories I was taking in.*** I was consuming a lot of calories but not much of it was nutritional. So all my body could do with it was store it as fat. It was hard to wrap my head around the fact that as fat as I was, I was still malnourished. So instead of burning fat for energy everything I ate mostly went straight to fat storage because the body uses ingested sugars first as energy rather than burn fat for energy. All because it takes longer for other nutrients to be broken down to be used as fuel the body makes use of the sugars eaten first. So these 800 calories per day was going to be of foods that my body could use and was going to be a step up (as far as my body was concerned) from the approximate 500 calories it was able to extract from a diet of junk food. The key was to get nutritional foods into my system that my body could use and do everything possible to boost my metabolism to melt the fat to use as energy instead of using refined sugar and carbohydrates as energy. *The most important thing I learned at the weight loss clinic was that out of all of the calories that I was eating my body was still* **undernourished**. Therefore my body was sending signals urging me to eat more. And of course I would eat more… eat more junk food. Thus, it was a vicious cycle that I was in. I'd spent the money on this program and I wanted it to work so I made the agreement to stick to it. You are not going to believe me when I tell you this, but I was **SO SICK OF EATING I DIDN'T KNOW WHAT TO DO**! Yes, you're reading right. I was **SO SICK OF EATING I DIDN'T KNOW WHAT TO DO**. A healthy eating plan for weight loss **does not call for starvation** it calls for **EATING. EATING** plenty of the **RIGHT KINDS OF FOOD**. Imagine my surprise at finding it difficult to consume 800 calories per day! For example, my new eating plan was one boiled egg, a turkey sausage patty, half a grapefruit and a ½ cup of coconut milk for breakfast which was about 300 calories. Whereas I was used to a coffee and a taco for breakfast which was about 800 calories. For lunch I was used to heavy lunches but many times I was very busy so I would grab a bag of chips and a 32 oz sweet tea—800 calories, but my new lunch was 4 ounces of chicken and a 1 ½ cup of spinach/kale mix with a lemon vinaigrette.—300 calories. Then being that I didn't have a real lunch by break time I'd have more chips, another tea and a candy bar—1200 calories vs. yogurt and ¼ c of nuts—200 calories. Then dinner would be a bacon cheeseburger with fries and another large sweet tea—1500 calories. My new dinner would be 4 oz. of beef with a cup of carrots and a cup of green beans—500 calories. There was a marked difference in the quantity of food for me to be healthy, versus the loaded calories with very few nutritional value in the small quantity of food that I had been eating. Then there is the frequency of eating that I'd never considered—I was told to not go more than four hours without eating whereas before I was used to going long stretches of time without eating which encourages the body to slow metabolism and store fat even more. I was just not used to eating so much food. I didn't want to risk getting sick so I had to work to get all the food in. I learned that this is why so many people use My Fitness Pal.com to record and monitor their eating and their exercise to keep track of it all. I found out the hard way that the software will not even store your information if you haven't eaten enough in a day. When it comes to weight loss, the overall calories consumed matter more than how often you eat but remember no two people are alike. So try to keep a steady frequency of eating.

I already knew that I hadn't been eating the right foods so I was glad that I was changing that but imagine my surprise when I realized that when it came to the right foods I had NOT been eating enough. This is a problem for many trying to lose weight. In an effort to reduce calorie intake, they reduce too much. So instead of increasing metabolism they end up slowing down metabolism more. So in spite of the fact that they are sticking to a plan they end up not getting the results they want. Your eating plan must include a sufficient amount of calories. Good caloric intake depends on sex, daily physical activity, age, current weight and weight loss goal. Using My Fitness Pal mine came up as 1840 calories. And I had no idea how difficult it would be to eat right until I had to put it into practice. But because of the agreement I made with myself I did, indeed, put it into practice. And I am so GLAD that I did.

Sufficient Nutrition Exercise

I hope that you can come to an understanding about getting sufficient nutrition. Make sure you're eating enough. As soon as you can wean yourself off the junk food. Go lean meaning abstinence from carbs and sugar and processed foods. Then your body cannot take a shortcut and use the carbs and sugars for energy it will be forced to melt the fat for energy. Complete the exercise below.

Write down what you typically eat in a day. Should be keeping a journal in My Fitness Pal by now so it should not be hard to take a look at the nutritional value in what you've been eating.

____

____

Next to each food item write down nutritional values of each one: Start with the **calories** (Use MyFitnessPal or use a search engine with key words "nutritional value of ________").
You should already **know how many calories you want in your meals** throughout the day. So make sure what you had planned, lines up with your actions.

____

____

Next look at how much **fat** (how much & what type, saturated, trans, **polyunsaturated—**), (Remember monounsaturated, polyunsaturated fat is good fat. **Limit the saturated fats and avoid Trans-fat as much as possible (10% of your caloric intake).** *Can consume up to 40% of caloric intake of the other three—not with junk food but meats, avocado, nuts, seeds and oils).*

____

____

____

Check the label on all processed foods, Especially notate how much **sodium** (*try to limit to 1500 mg per day*),

____

____

How much **added carbs/sugars** (Broken down into total carbs, fiber and sugar. **Limit to 25 grams of carbs and 5gms of sugar.** You may subtract the grams of fiber from the number of total carbs.

____

____

____

Lastly, note the **nutrient type** of your foods (protein, carb, and fruit/veggie). (**Recommended max protein—56 grams max per day for sedentary man and 46 grams max per day for sedentary woman.** Notate vitamins and minerals- fiber, potassium, vitamin A or C, etc.?)

____

____

____

____

Did you find a lot of nutritional value in your meals? Or not so much? How much sugar or sodium?

____

____

____

What is the total of calories for what you typically eat in a day? Are you eating enough?

____

____

____

How much of your calorie intake is in what you're drinking?

____

____

____

Any way to substitute high caloric/fatty/sugary foods or drinks for those better for your health?

____

____

____

Look up the nutritional value of what you usually eat at your favorite restaurants on My Fitness Pal and make some decisions about what's going to be your go-to choices from the menu whenever you visit them in the future.

What's the nutritional value in your favorite snack? Make some decisions about how often you're going to allow this treat. Can you substitute?

Example – Nutritional Value of My Typical Breakfast

BFST- 2 egg omelet with 2 TBSP spicy turkey sausage, pico di gallo and spinach

2 eggs: 150 calories, fat 9 gr (3 sat, 2 poly, 4 mono), sodium 140mg, carb/sugar 0, protein 12g

Tbsp of butter: 102 calories, fat11.52 g (7 sat, .4 poly, 3 mono)

Spicy turkey sausage: 44 calories, fat 3 gr (sat.5, .6 poly, .7 mono) sodium 168mg, carb/sugar 0, protein 5 g,

Pico di gallo: calories 10, fat 0, sodium 0, sugar 0

½ c spinach: calories 7, fat 0, sodium 0, sugar 0, Vit A, Vit C, 167 potassium

Eating for Nutritional Value Journal

Journal your thoughts and experiences regarding making the switch to choosing foods for their nutritional value

____

____

____

____

____

____

____

____

____

____

Breaking the Chains of a Sugar Addiction

A huge part of my transition was switching from eating junky foods to eating healthy foods. To stick to eating healthy I had to break my habit of my love for sugary foods. Research about whether or not sugar is addictive is inconclusive. But for me I know with a certainty that I had an addiction to sugar because I would never go home without making sure cookies, candy, chips and something sweet to drink was there. If I knew I was all out, I had to make a stop for my snacks. Now in regards to my meals, I was totally out of control. Examples of my meals was that of burgers and fries, fried chicken with a biscuit and more fries. I loved pizza and chili-cheese hot dogs with slushes and tots. There's no way to get through San Antonio without tacos and barbeque. All these different foods were in heavy rotation from day to day and week after week. When the budget was tight I had spaghetti, lasagna, chicken Alfredo and chili mac three to four times a week. For most of my meals, I ate out and then I always topped it off with sugary snacks. If I could live off of chips and sweet tea that would be all I'd ever eat. I could never go into a store and come out without buying some sort of treat—cookies, candy or ice cream. So when I cut sugar from my diet I had to suffer through it. I would sweat profusely. I had headaches all the time and my stomach turned with queasiness most days. I would fall asleep at any time and almost anywhere. I was lightheaded and dizzy and often had to lay down in the middle of the day. But not for long because I always felt antsy. It was like I didn't know what to do with myself. It reminded me of Jamie Foxx as he played the role of Ray Charles in the movie **Ray,** the biopic about the legendary singer, songwriter. When Ray quit drugs cold turkey, he rolled in the bed for days. Well that's how I felt without sugar. To break the sugar addiction I stuck to the plan given to me. Often times actually sobbing for the beloved foods I refused to eat. I would munch on ice, have a peppermint or chew gum (My favorites were Birthday cake by Project 7 and Artic Chill by Dentyne). Then I learned that this could have been easier to get through with a little sugar water. From my church group I learned about putting a cup of orange juice (or 2 oz. of maple syrup or honey) in 32 ounces of water to sip on as needed throughout the day and that helped a lot. I would get on my laptop and do searches for what happens to the body when we eat sugar and I'd read the articles or reports. Once you read one search about health, there will be 5 new "tips" or links waiting for you the next time you turn on your computer. So that helped to keep my mind occupied. When you learn what you're doing is detrimental to your body, you can make better choices. I focused on how I didn't want to waste the money I spent on the program so I concentrated on eating only foods on the list they gave me. I found fruit and nuts to be the most satisfying to substitute my favorites. I hadn't wanted to take the appetite suppressants prescribed to me but I finally caved in and they helped with cravings and nausea. I had retired from my career of 18 years as a mortgage processor at a financial services company in December of 2015 and had decided to take some time off to get my master's degree in Organizational Development before re-entering the work force. I was glad that I was not working while my body de-toxed from sugar. One day it got so bad that it scared me. I was thinking maybe my blood sugar was too low. I checked and it was 154 which is relatively high. When I told the doctor at the weight loss clinic about my experiences she told me that I described the symptoms of hypoglycemia (low blood sugar) and for my body to think 154mg/dl, was low my average was likely 250 or more on a regular basis prior to changing my diet which is a really dangerous place to be health wise. From the nutrition clinic I was sent to by my endocrinologist I'd learned that for someone without diabetes, a fasting blood sugar level upon awakening should be between 70–99 Milligrams per deciliter of blood (mg/dl). Two hours after meals blood sugar should be less than 140 mg/dl. Those are the normal numbers for someone without diabetes. For someone who has diabetes, the usual aim is to keep fasting blood sugar levels between 80–130 mg/dl and levels 1–2 hours after meals under 180. So the weight loss clinic physician and I were both glad to see that I had the determination of mind to break the chains of this sugar addiction and to make this change a life-style change and to never go back to the way that I used to eat. After about a two weeks my body eventually calmed down and I adjusted. I just had to tough it out. I drank a lot of water and got plenty of rest. It's all about choice. Once I made up my mind, my actions followed through with the firm decision. I hope you can use the exercises below to make some firm decisions about your bad habits that are keeping you from getting fit.

Break the Chains Exercise

We have to eat, right? So how can we be addicted to food? Take this quiz to find out.
Have you ever wanted to stop eating something and found you couldn't?____

____

Do you eat differently in front of other people than you do by yourself?____

____

Do you severely restrict food intake?

____

____

Do you exercise excessively?

____

____

Do you binge? Or do you binge and purge?

____

____

Have you spent years dieting—losing and gaining weight, ending up   gaining   more   weight   than   when started?___________________________

____

____

If you answered yes to any of these questions, then yes; you have food issues. If you're not able to break the cycle and gain control working through the resources in this book, I recommend that you seek   a   professional   that   can   help   you   transform.

____

____

There is a solution. You're already on the path if you've been doing the exercises at the end of each chapter in this book. It takes the following:

Write down your food plan. This way you know what, when and how much you are going to eat. If not sure, you may use the information in the chapter exercises entitled My Twist on Professor Haub's Plan.

Know your boundaries. Your boundaries to work towards is a sufficient amount exercise and to meet calorie intake goals.

Choose exercise that yields 500 calories burned daily. (Hopefully you were able to go to the Physical Activity Calorie Counter located at American Council of Exercise at www. Acefitness.org. See chapter entitled Know your Chemistry) Take a look at the calories burned in doing different exercises to make some decisions about what you'd like to do for your physical activity).

Know the maximum calories you want to eat each day. Hopefully you have been able to figure out your Basal Metabolic Rate (BMR) and have calculated a 1/3 of that amount. And that amount is your daily caloric goal. Do NOT just estimate the calories. You must weigh and measure portions. So if you haven't done these two exercises do them now so you'll know your boundaries.

____

____

Review the agreements that you've made daily. Review your agreements every morning and every night. Put them in your phone for emergencies.

____

____

Abstinence. This is going to take a commitment to abstain from sugar to let go of addictive eating. I did this for a time and somehow I have it under control, but some people will have a need to stay away from sugar forever as a recovering alcoholic would abstain from drinking.

____

____

Self-care. Appreciate your body and yourself right now at the weight that you are by having gratitude that you're making strides towards good health.

____

____

Support. This addiction is a disease of isolation. Find a support group. Find an accountability partner. Have someone who will take your call any time day or night to talk you off the ledge of a food craving or compulsion. Those who are addicted to food are often self-centered, so volunteer, reach out and extend a helping hand to someone other than yourself.

____

____

This is also going to take acknowledging a greater power. I'm not trying to force my religion or my faith on you, but I am a believer because I know that I didn't speak myself into existence and it is with certainty that I have little say in when I will leave this earthly plain. When I was adrift, I connected with the spiritual side of me and today I have love, peace and joy that's unshakeable. No matter what comes, I know that I am not alone. There's a spiritual side of you that contains a portion of the greater power. And the only way out of your issues with food is to connect with it. It means quiet time. Defend your mind by stopping all negative chatter. It means loving and coaching yourself to heal and forgive. It means helping others. Explore prayer, meditation and scripture reading—start at The Book of Psalms

It takes Strategy to Stick to a Meal Plan

I pretty much knew I would have a problem sticking to 800 calories per day so I ordered a meal plan from Dr. Marlene Merritt, the creator of the Blood Pressure Solution. (Merritt, 2015) It's a really neat subscription. Every week they send a meal plan that includes a grocery list and recipes. You go to the store and get all the items on the list and you're all set for 3 tasty, healthy meals per day to get you through the entire week. She sends a guide that explains why she's incorporating the different items in the recipes—lean proteins, good fats, leafy vegetables and foods to avoid. Well, I had a problem because this lasted about two weeks. I started receiving the meal plans but I wasn't cooking. Why? The problem with meal plans for me was getting through the store without buying stuff *not* on my list. Going to the grocery store was extremely difficult for me and caused great anxiety in me because of all the temptations to buy the wrong foods. I got to where I would go into the store and get spinach, carrots and cucumbers in the produce section, get Oscar Mayer turkey and chicken deli meats, frozen fully cooked chicken and beef fajita strips and eggs then run to the register to get out of there praying the whole time that I could get through the line without succumbing to the impulse buying of soda, chips or candy on the way out. My goal was to work my way to eating meats that were not processed but that was the best strategy I could devise at the time. But the more I got results, the easier it was to change. I'm stronger today because I allow myself a treat day as well as one small treat per day for one of my snack. So I can get through the store by reminding myself that I can hold off until the scheduled time. I've learned to restrict myself to 30 grams of carbs per day—so once a day I can have a sweet treat—like a few squares of 70% dark chocolate (after a while I developed the discipline for one M&M "fun size" package of candy. There are some really good cookie crisps. My favorite is Crunchy Cookie Chips by Hannah Max Baking, Oatmeal raisin or salted peanut butter are really good, because I can have 5 of them or Chips Ahoy Thins® – (or 10 on workout day!) Sometimes I crave something starchy like a baked potato or baked sweet potato and I use my 30 grams of carbs on that. Or I can use my carbohydrate allowance for bread to make a sandwich or small serving of pasta or flour tortilla to make a breakfast taco or taco shells for taco salad or even chips and salsa or DORITOS®! I also discovered that shopping at Whole Foods or Sprouts is a better option for me when I *am* feeling vulnerable to temptation because everything there is good for me.

The other thing I learned through this process is that it takes strategy to stick to a meal plan. This whole process may involve going through your office and the house and throwing out all the tempting foods you do not need to eat right now. It may take having a talk with family and friends about how you are going to stop eating poorly; you will limit dining out and drinking alcoholic beverages; and need their support in this lifestyle change. Planning dinner may involve Crockpot cooking or cooking the major portions of your meals— perhaps the meats, on weekends. You have to be prepared with food packs in order to have healthy snacks in between meals— just like it's done for a toddler, you can do it for yourself. I often keep an apple, a box of raisins or a small package of nuts in my purse. Also, when I started this I knew it would be challenging but I agreed to make the commitment to stick to the plan because I needed to become a better me. I remember thinking if this was for family or friends I'd do it. I'll do anything and everything to keep a commitment to or for someone else. So why not do for myself what I would do for others. It was time to stop putting myself on the backburner. This is how I was able to come to an agreement that I could be at peace with. I never say that I can or I cannot have a particular food. I always say *"I can have anything I want*, except I CHOOSE *NOT* TO EAT THOSE THINGS THAT I KNOW WILL SET ME BACK." I further agreed that *if there was anything that I really wanted to eat, I could go ahead and allow myself to eat it, I would just get the smallest portion available and would take slow bites or sips, pausing between intakes so that I could then know to stop upon satisfaction.* I have found that I rarely eat more than half of a child-sized portion of a treat that I've been craving yet I'm satisfied but haven't totally wrecked my weight loss plan. Somewhere I learned that a person has to eat 1000 extra calories than they use in a day to gain a pound. So if a person hasn't eaten an additional 1000 calories yet has gained 2 to 4 pounds it is likely water weight (or something other than fat). So if what you are eating outside of your food plan is a few bites or a small portion of a treat it shouldn't derail your whole weight loss program. One of my favorite treats is to get two Chips Ahoy! Thins and put one 1 TBSP of H-E-B Creamy Creations® 1905 Vanilla Ice Cream in the middle. It's the perfect snack without getting you too far off track. Just be sure to limit the frequency and quantity of treats allowed. The other thing I've learned is that after getting used to eating a certain way I wind up with a headache, stomachache or actual displeasure that a treat didn't taste as good as it used to. Then I do not have to have a game plan to avoid certain foods, I don't even want them.

Something else I learned to do when I go to a fast food place is choose which carb—bread, potatoes, sugary drink or desert. So if I'm at Dairy Queen, I'll have tacos or a salad because I know I want a mini Blizzard. And if I go to Chick-Fil-A, I'm deciding am I going to be good and have a salad? Do I eat a kids meal so that I can have a little of it all? Do I want a sandwich or nuggets? If I have a regular sized sandwich then I get a side salad and unsweetened tea. If I really want waffle fries then I'll get tenders and unsweetened tea, but not a sandwich to avoid the bread. Yes, that's right I drink unsweetened tea without any sweetener. If there is a mix up and I get sweetened tea, I get it corrected or give it to my husband because I can't even drink sweetened tea nowadays. So many junk food items have lost their power over me. Hallelujah!

The other thing is when I'm allowing myself a treat and it's just so-so, I don't finish it because it's not worth the calories.

Plan Your Strategy Exercise

Use the exercise below to formulate strategies to keep your agreements towards fitness.

Getting through the grocery store. Know where all your usual items are located. In most stores the outer perimeter is where you find everything you need-- produce, meats, dairy and frozen. Shop at stores like Whole Foods and Sprouts if there's room in your budget. Arrange for your spouse, adult children or a trusted friend to shop for you and buy exactly what you have on the list until you get past any addictions and you're strong enough to avoid falling into temptation. Once your weight is going in the right direction and you see that sticking to your meal plan is paying off, you'll be able to resist and shop for yourself.

Go through the house and throw out all the stuff you know will not be a part of your meal plan.

Go through the office and throw out all the stuff you know will not be a part of your meal plan.

Plan breakfast. Are you going to eat breakfast at home before you leave the house, take it to work or eat at work—which choice invites the least amount of temptation? If you're eating at work, is there a lean option for breakfast at work but doesn't cause you to be stray to the wrong foods.

Plan lunch. Are you taking your lunch to work, eating at the work cafeteria or going out for lunch? If not bringing my own lunch, how will you stick to my eating plan?

Plan dinner. For dinner if you eat meat, choose meats that cook in 30 minutes or you can think about preparing at least the meats on the weekend so that you can get dinner on the table swiftly during the week. One thing I love to do is collect crockpot recipes so I can put everything in the slow cooker when I get up in the morning and let it cook all day so that dinner is ready in a timely manner. I like the following books for help with meal preparation: *Meal Prep Cookbook for Beginners* by Nancy Crews and *The Make Ahead Kitchen* by Annalise Thompson.

Go over the menus of your favorite places to eat (fast food types as well as sit down dining) and choose 2 or 3 entrees that you can select from whenever you visit that will not unravel your fitness progress.

Work to get family/friends/coworkers/partners on board with food plan to keep from planning separate dishes.

Intersections. Know your danger zones. It is extremely important to sit down and identify the intersections where the new habits need to replace the bad habits. So that you'll know to shore yourself up when you're in a spot that's full of temptation. Then plan tactics to get past the danger zone without wrecking yourself. The intersections to start with are **every time you eat** and **every time you shop**.

Eating. As mentioned in a previous chapter plan your meals and prepare them ahead to avoid eating out of turn.

For situations that trigger snacking, munching and grazing, like watching television or going to the movies, plan and portion out what you're going to eat. I tend to eat Skinny Girl popcorn at home and a pickle at the movies.

Every time you get ready to put something in your mouth, FREEZE; ask yourself **are you really hungry?; AND is this on your plan**?

Practice mindful eating to avoid emotional eating. Remember that it's better to confront fears and frustrations than it is to feed them.

Review your commitments each morning AND night to stick to your plan daily to avoid following your plan all week only to blow it as you go through social events over the weekend.

To avoid eating on the run before you head out review which meal times you're going to go through while out. Take your prepared food with you if at all possible. Don't be afraid to care for yourself just like you would for a toddler. If not able to take your food with you plan to eat at a place that prepares healthy dishes. Always have a healthy snacks in your purse.

For shopping, every time you get ready to go into a store review your commitment. Agree on a budget, what you are going to buy and what you are NOT going to buy. Put your commitment agreement in your phone where you can easily access it for review. Every store, even a hardware store has goodies. You know where the goodies are in the store so avoid those aisles. If you're going grocery shopping try going to a store like Whole Foods until you gain some control because they do not have candy, chips and soda around the register when you're trying to check out.

Strategy Journal

Write out the strategies that you planned. Write your experiences. Did they work to keep you on the straight and narrow? If not, how did you revise them or what's your alternate plan?

____

____

____

____

____

____

____

____

____

____

____

____

____

____

____

____

Eureka!!

Seeking a way to get nutrients in me I found this guide by David Andrews entitled *The Type II Diabetes Destroyer System* (Andrews, 1976) and he did a really good job coaching me to better nutrition and he introduced me to Troy Adashun, certified nutrition expert and personal trainer, and they helped me to understand how processed foods were impeding my progress. David Andrews and Troy Adashun both recommended different types of smoothies but I didn't like how they turned out. I didn't want to have to go and buy a whole bunch of stuff to make a different smoothie every day. I wanted one smoothie that I could make the same way every day that had everything in it that I needed. But I didn't like the taste of the different spices like turmeric and cayenne in a vanilla or chocolate shake. One day when I was taste testing, something about the earthiness reminded me of tea. So I decided to make a tea with the ingredients and EUREKA!! That was the key. The plan was to drink the tea three times a day but I managed only twice a day and the results were staggering. I gave some to my husband and because of the vinegar, lemon and cayenne (I like extra) he described it as "fire water". To better define the tea and separate the name from any possible reference to alcohol or group of people, I added the distinction of fat melting and the descriptive of tea instead of water to the title because it is in fact a tea and that's what the tea appears to do—the fat just melts off the body. But folks started calling it Trena Tea so I ran with that. With the fat sculpting clinic I went from 230 to 214 when I found the tea and got down to 210. After another four weeks using high intensity exercise, full body exercise and including the tea on every other week I went from 210 to 204 pounds. I made it to my goal of losing 40 pounds. The most important thing for me was not necessarily the pounds I lost but that the fat in my middle just melted away and my clothes look better on me. I am not sure how many inches because I didn't record my waist measurements previously.

Grow Your Way Out

As you look over your life, I'm certain you'll find that every problem (no matter how painful) is there to help you grow. There are no mistakes. Every situation that happens to you is necessary for growth. There's a thought process I use to keep moving forward. I call it the **TRHS** (my initials) **Revelation** (life-truth revealed usually through growing pains) **Theory**. I use it any time I have a problem because I want that problem to disappear as quickly as possible. And it's not going anywhere until I receive the seed of revelation that is there all wrapped up in the problem for me to uncover.

Here's how it works. First you address the emotion. Feel the anger, worry, anxiety, fear, distress, embarrassment etc. Let it flow freely and as soon as there is a break from the pain set your despair aside long enough to think about what you could possibly gain from the situation. You either need to learn a **life-lesson**, perfect a **life-change** (stop doing something, start doing something or change the way you do things—permanently, in the way that a butterfly cannot go back to being a caterpillar), complete a **life-task** that has to do with your overall purpose in life, and finally, **mature---** gain insight, clarity and change the way you perceive things so that you make smarter moves, ready for the next level. We go through growing pains to gain one or all four aspects of growth; all for the purpose of preparing us to operate on another plain. So to be fit if we know what we need to do yet we are not successful in achieving and maintaining our fitness goals, we have to start at the beginning. Acknowledging that we each must figure out what we individually need to extract from the vast array of fitness material out there, and incorporate it into our lives to get the results we want. If you want things to change, you've got to change.

So let's apply the revelation theory to fitness. Your goal is to go through all the aspects of fitness and determine what works for you and your goals. If you can **figure the keys** to weight loss for you, that's a huge (lesson). Then once you learn your lesson(s), you **become clear about what you need to start, stop or change**. To make it stick, you then **identify the intersections** where you've been taking the wrong action and replace it with the new action (change). So the key to change is to 1) do a good job identifying the intersection of pitfalls 2) **develop the correct strategies** that keep you from succumbing to things that take you off track 3) **replace the old action with the new action** (change). You may do so well that this may turn into a life task for you. My quest turned into a life-task to write the tea book and manufacture Trena Tea (purpose). I do not know what's in store for you. But I do know that the way you approach and do one thing is the way you do everything. Think about the things in life that you do well and you'll realize that it's because you paid attention to the details. Somewhere along the way you've missed the details in taking care of yourself. But conquer this huge mountain and you will begin to apply these same skills to overcome the other challenges in your life. Right now somewhere in your daily routine you are being childish--not active enough; don't know what a portion is; eat when NOT hungry; won't stop eating when full; addicted to certain foods; only eat one real meal a day; love to eat; not eating enough; not drinking enough water; too much snacking; use eating to cope with other issues etc… in terms of weight management. So the only way out is to *grow* your way out. Everything that you learn, change and complete will mature you to be able to handle the next set of challenges life presents (growth). Somebody say "Amen for growth and maturity!"

Beware of Dream Killers

Here is some information that I hope will help you with the negativity of others to make it on your journey. This was a tip that evolved into its own section because so much of our food issues are born of our relationship issues. Stay away from dream killers. Guard your dreams. Protect your dreams. Be careful who you share your dreams and goals with. Not everyone is worthy of hearing your dreams. For example, you will find out that some people you can share the reason why you're avoiding certain foods or drinks and with others you will learn that they can't handle the fact that you've decided to be firm about your fitness goals. To them you may want to learn to say "No thanks, I'm not hungry right now." or "Got so busy running around today that I had to eat before I got here, I'm stuffed now… I'm good... I don't need anything." Why open up yourself to be a target for the misplaced insecurities of others? I've learned that we teach people how to treat us. In every situation that I've found myself feeling mistreated, it was because others learned that it was acceptable to treat me that way. I've also learned to stop looking to others for validation. I had to learn to consult someone who's been successful at what I'm attempting to achieve. I learned to carefully search myself against those who have gone before me to determine whether my ideals were sound and ready to launch or in need of more preparation. I say to you stop looking outside yourself to others for approval. Your dream is for you and often times others cannot see where you're going or how you're going to make it. There's no support. They are going by their own experiences. Well their experience does not have to be yours. I saw this expression on the Internet recently, "You can't make someone be ready for what you're ready for and you're not obligated to wait around for them to make up their mind." *And yes, the odds may be stacked against you in terms of reaching your goals but listen to the advice given if for no other reason than to come up with a strategy to bridge the gap over the troubled waters they "foresee".* That's right, use the negativity to create a better success plan; so that you don't succumb to pitfalls along the way. The last thing you need is for those things said by naysayers to come into fruition. If you do not go for your goals you end up making somebody else's dream come true.

Mental Strength

Talk less, do more. Do the work on yourself so that you have the right mental attitude to get where you're trying to go. *Realize that you are not where you want to be because you are missing the insight it takes to get there. You must humble yourself and stop being a "know it all" and become an investigator to get where you want to be.* If you want things to get better, you've got to get better. You can't change your life without changing your mind. Here I want to encourage you to think about what you're internally speaking over your life.

In this regard, you cannot cheat. You must do the work— you need to be the best YOU that you can be; you must do the exploration to become a SKILLED MASTER, an expert, at whatever it is you're trying to accomplish; you need to DEVELOP A PLAN from your research and you need to TAKE ACTION. You need to do that action **with consistency—*long enough*** to get results.

YOU-- I have found that to be the best "self" in life we must be **graceful** (poised/debonair) this keeps us from behaving inappropriately; be **anchored** (grounded in a belief system—for me that's keeping my one on one relationship with God through song, prayer and scripture-- staying honest with self, maintaining life as it is even while chasing after dreams); be **transformational** (Make the changes required to get to the next level); be **empowered** (NO LIMIT—stop telling yourself what you cannot do… give yourself permission to do what you CAN do NOW and then layer on more refined action as you *learn* more and be **dauntless** (Don't back down. Pinpoint the places of change. Have the self-control to stick to your game plan by being organized enough to do the new habits instead of the old ones at those point + plan what you're going to do with your time so you don't waste it + be courageous (do it afraid) + be resilient) --*I like to use the acronym GATED because possessing these characteristics locks failure out.*

MASTER YOUR SKILL -- Then for your project, do the research. Study what's online (review with a grain of salt because you can't believe everything on the Internet); see every video, read every book, report, article and journal about your subject. No one should know more about the thing you're trying to achieve than you. Become a sponge and soak up all the information you can find regarding your field and become a master in your field. Go to workshops. Interview and network with people who are successful where you're trying to go. Decide what you're keeping or throwing out from what you've learned. Determine what you can expand on to take the existing information to another level.

MAKE A PLAN-- Develop a plan from what you've learned. Try using S.M.A.R.T—Specific, Significant, Stretching; Measurable, Meaningful, Motivational; Attainable, Action-oriented, Achievable; Realistic, Relevant, Rewarding and Time-based, Tangible, Trackable. Get a calendar and schedule what you're going to do and when. Putting a deadline on your plan makes it a true goal rather than a fantasy.

ACTION-- All of the work means nothing if you do not take action. You have to at least TRY to reach your goal. Then go back and review your actions against your plans—that my friends is called *ACCOUNTABILITY*.

Sometimes we are not where we want to be because we are in our own way because we lack clarity about what we really want. Other times we have such limiting thoughts—the way we think of things we would like and then we say to ourselves "if only it could really happen". Then other times we hold such a stubborn insistence that things unfold in a certain way so we fail to maintain mental focus when the view on the horizon doesn't look how we'd planned. Mental focus is holding a clear view of your desires steadfast in your mind no matter what things look like. And here's how you gain mental strength. Listen for the small, still voice so that you will know for certain the RIGHT THING to do. **If you're not at peace, don't make a move.** *Do everything that is within your* *power to do,* **then maintain a positive outlook until something happens.** Please, please get out of the way. Go with the flow. Let it unfold. Continue to hone and master your skills so that you'll be prepared to walk through, when the door of opportunity is opened. You absolutely cannot worry and you cannot fret because negativity brings more negativity. Coach to yourself using these words:

"Whatever the outcome is, it is… And it will be good."

Do not allow anyone—partner, family, friends or enemies to disturb your vision or to be effective in causing you to give up on your goals.

Have Faith

Finally, you must have faith. See it. Believe it. Picture yourself receiving and enjoying the culmination of your weight loss dreams. **If you can't see yourself in possession of the body shape you desire I don't know why you would expect to receive it.** Sometimes we have to bring up our self-value to picture the unthinkable happening for us. "Why not us?" Who says magical things only happen to the "Oprahs" in the world. If you find yourself doubting, start with believing small things adjusting your thinking to a picture you *can* believe and then repeat. The more you exercise your faith, the stronger it gets. Also, change the negative internal chatter that says, "Someday" to "I'm open to receive all that has been planned for me." Fear, worry and anxiety are the opposite of faith. So we must banish away the emotions that rise up with anxious thoughts. I refuse to add to the adversary's pleasure by revealing how deep the blows of life strike. Don't fret or stress about it. **Find a place of peace**, (exchange objecting and rejecting the circumstances to accepting things as they are with the realization that the power of God is greater than them all and something good will come of the turmoil), **picture it** (Call those things that are not as if they were) and **release it** (forget about it). To help me banish worrisome thoughts like "Lord, *please, please, please* let this project come through for me!" I do what David did. I encourage myself in the Lord. I say things like, "I believe this is what You want me to do. You've equipped me. You've empowered me. I'm going to do my very best and I'm going to trust You to do the rest to get me to the next level. Give me the boldness I need to overcome my fears, challenges and setbacks so that I become all that You've created me to be."

I have to catch myself—because if I'm worrying about it after I've prayed about it that means that I'm *NOT* TRUSTING God to come through for me. Then I'm being offensive to God by questioning the provision He has made for me. If you know the thoughts God thinks towards you are, "…thoughts of peace and not of evil, to give you an expected end" Jer 29:11 and other translations state "plans to prosper you and not to harm you, plans to give you hope and a future" then you know that your job is to calm yourself, maintain the expectancy of a blessing as you hold on until the change comes. The truth of the matter is if we do not believe it we *cannot* receive it. Jesus said *Therefore I say unto you, what things so ever ye desire, when ye pray, believe that ye receive them, and ye shall have them.* Mark 11: 24. So then I remind myself that I've already prayed about it, so now from this point on I'm not going to keep going back and picking up this burden. I'm leaving it with God every time the thought tries to return, then I push every negative thought away with scriptures and say *Stand still and see the salvation* (deliverance) *of the Lord*…Exodus 14: 13. I follow that up with *The battle is not yours but God's* II Chronicles 20:15. Then I remember that *all things are working together for good*… Romans 8:28. And *God is able to make all grace abound toward you, that ye always having all sufficiency in all things, may abound to every good work,* II Corinthians 9:8. Let us pray.

Father God,

Help us keep the faith and be motivated to take good care of our bodies. We ask Your help in carrying through with our commitments to exercise, eat right and get sufficient rest. Free us from all pain, relationship ills and stress that's compelling us to eat out of turn. Help us to break the chains of all food addictions. Please guide us to know the best information, books and research to take care of ourselves and get some real results. Help us to resist procrastination and stay driven to endure until we reach our goals. We pray that the changes we make will be lifestyle changes so that we may never go back to that which we were. We know You are able to do exceedingly abundantly above all that we ask or think. We ask that You give your children the strength to continue to look to the hills from which cometh all our help. Please touch, heal, deliver and make us free. In the name of the One that gave it all, Amen.

New Beginnings

Now make no mistake this was only a beginning because I have a long way to go. My blood glucose levels are much improved. My blood sugar is in normal range most mornings. My doctor found substitutes for the other two medications but I no longer need them. When I drop 10 more pounds I will have a BMI that's normal. And the tea is a huge re-setting strategy to bridge all the gaps that I'll face along the way.

And I'm hoping you can use this information to get you passed any stumbling blocks you face. When I couldn't follow the regimen that had been given to me and I was stalled at one particular weight for weeks and was tempted to throw in the towel, I started taking the tea. And because I started getting results I had the discipline to stick to my meal plans. I learned that 1600 to 1800 calories per day is a healthy range with 10,000 steps per day or 30 minutes of high intensity interval training or full bodied isometric exercises using as many large muscles as possible did the trick to jump start my metabolism. But that it was self-care and very much okay to start where I was and work my way toward my goal. I'm now able to go into the grocery store and not be tempted by all the treats available. I hope that you find some information in this book useful.

If you decide to try the tea, I would love to see your before and after photos along with a brief story of how things worked out for you. I'm on Facebook at Trena Tea, you may inquire about the Trena Tea as well as upload photos there.

References

Ainsworth, B.E., Haskell, W.L., Hermann SD, Meckes N., Bassett

Jr D.R, Tudo Glover M.C., Leon, A.S. The Compendium

of Physical Activities Tracking Guide. Healthy Lifestyles

Research CenterAinsworth BE, H. W.-L.-G. (2011,

August). *Compendium of Physical Activities*. Retrieved

from

https://sites.google.com/site/compendiumofphysicalactiviti

es/

American Council of Exercise, A. (2017, July 25). Retrieved from

acefitness.org:

https://www.acefitness.org/acefit/healthy_living_tools_cont

ent.aspx?id=1

Andrews, D. (1976). Type II Diabetes Destroyer.

Coffey-Meyer, K. (Director). (2015). *30 Minutes to Fitness:*

Muscle Up Lift 2B Fit with Kelly Coffey-Meyer [Motion

Picture].

Freedhoff, Y. (2014). *The Diet Fix: Why Diets Fail and How to Make Yours Work*. New York City: Potter/TenSpeed/Harmony.

Guise, S. (2013). *Mini Habits: Small Habits, Bigger Results*. Stephen Guise.

Hughes, K. (2012, April 16). *Cooper Institute*. Retrieved from https://www.cooperinstitute.org/2012/04/met-minutes-a-simple-common-value-to-track-exercise-progress/

Kiczek, P. (2017, May). *NJ2NY50- The Big Walk*. Retrieved from http://nj2ny50.org/calorie-estimator-how-many-calories-do-you-burn-walking

Lockhart, E. (2014, April 8). *Active Beat.com*. Retrieved from http://www.activebeat.com/diet-nutrition/8-pieces-of-mindful-eating-wisdom/3/

McDougall, A. (2015, October 9). *Livestrong.com*. Retrieved from http://www.livestrong.com/article/330657-how-many-miles-do-i-need-to-walk-a-day-to-lose-75-pounds/

McGraw, P. (2003). *The Ulimate Weight Solution: The 7 Keys to Weight Loss Freedom*. New York, NY: Simon and Schuster.

Merritt, M. D. (2015). *Control Your Blood Pressure Naturally.*

Primal Health L.P.

Michaels, J. (Director). (2014). *Jillian Michaels Beginner Shred*

[Motion Picture].

Park, M. (2010, November 8). *CNN Health.* Retrieved from

Twinkie Diet Helps Nutrition Professor Lose 27 Pounds:

http://www.cnn.com/2010/HEALTH/11/08/twinkie.diet.pro

fessor/index.html

Robbins, M. (2014). *Nothing Changes Until You Do: A Guide to*

Self-Compassion and Getting Out of Your Own Way. Hay

House.

Sansone (Director). (2012). *Leslie Sansone: Just Walk-- Ultimate 5*

Day Walk Plan [Motion Picture].

Sansone, L. (Director). (2014). *Leslie Sansone: Just Walk-- Walk*

Off Fat Fast: Fat Burning Walks [Motion Picture].

Smith, Ian K. (2012). *Shred: The Revolutionary Diet: 6 Weeks 4*

Inches 2 Sizes. New York: St Martin's Press.

Solo, S. (2014, August 29). *Real Simple.com*. Retrieved from

     https://www.realsimple.com/health/nutrition-diet/weight-

     loss/busting-10-diet-myths

Steen, J. (2016, November 9). *Austrailian Huffington Post*.

     Retrieved from

     http:/www.huffingtonpost.com.au/2016/11/09/we-found-

     out-if-it-really-takes-20-minutes-to-feel-full/

Walters, R. (2016, April 27). *inbodyusa.com*. Retrieved from

     https://www.inbodyusa.com/blogs/inbodyblog/99465793-

     what-walking-10-000-steps-does-and-doesn-t-do-for-you